Eggshells

AND

Elephants

My Cancer Journey Thus Far

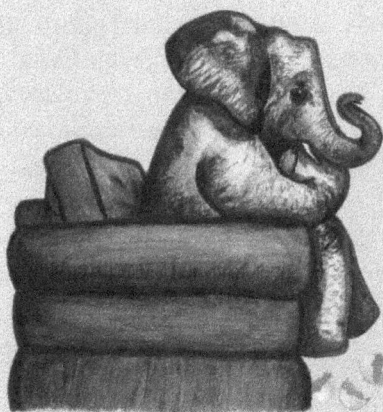

By **Jane Freund**

FREUNDSHIP
PRESS

Positively influencing lives through friendship, communication, and education.

ISBN: 978-0-9839957-8-4

Published by Freundship Press, LLC
PO Box 9171
Boise, ID 83707
info@freundshippress.com
www.freundshippress.com

DEDICATION

This book is dedicated to my paternal great-grandparents, Alois and Marie Goldmann, who are two of the most courageous people I never met. They made the ultimate sacrifice sending their only descendant, my dad, to America to escape the atrocities of the Holocaust. The Goldmanns were ultimately murdered at Auschwitz.

ABOUT THE AUTHOR

Jane Freund's first stated career goal was as a pre-schooler when she announced to her mother that she was going to be a pink elephant trainer. Jane ultimately chose another career path and taught communication for ten years at Boise State University in Boise, ID. Then, she left to form Freundship Press and to write, publish and speak on a full-time basis. Most recently, Jane conquered thyroid cancer. "Eggshells and Elephants – My Cancer Journey Thus Far" is the tenth book she has written or co-written.

Jane's other current work is titled "The Girl Who Had a Big Adventure – Cancer, Chemo & Cupcakes" which was written by Stacia Mers, an eight-year-old who conquered brain cancer. Jane had the privilege of co-authoring that book which is written by a kid for a kid (with a little help from an adult).

If you want to know more about Jane, read this book as pieces of her life story are peppered throughout the pages. You can reach Jane at jane@janefreund.com.

ACKNOWLEDGEMENTS

Cancer is like a library full of all sorts of different kinds of books. Some books are nonfiction: true stories full of facts and other information. Other volumes are fiction: tales which are made up and did not occur. Some books are romantic full of love, sadness, anger and other emotions. Still other books are humorous and make the readers laugh, smile and otherwise see the funny parts to life. The point of some books is how-to as instruction is the focus. A library can also contain books that are biographical telling either the author's or somebody else's life story.

This book is most definitely NOT fiction or romantic at least in terms of finding love. If that is what you are looking for, I suggest a good love story kind of movie or a Robin Lee Hatcher book. However this book is certainly a combination of nonfiction, autobiography, how-to, humor and other emotions. My cancer was and, although removed, still remains a very real part of my life. Through this book, I aim to give you a very realistic look at what happened to me from diagnosis through surgery to treatment and finally to life on the other side of cancer. Simply put, I stared death down and death blinked.

But I have made this journey far from alone and thus I want to acknowledge those who have helped me through this life-changing experience:

To my physicians Drs. Leslie Nona, Todd Rudstad and Richard Christensen and their teams: thank you for taking me through the process from funky blood test result through diagnosis, surgery and treatment to life forever with Synthroid.

To JoEllen, Kim, Kris, Linda, and Lori: thank you for giving me your brutally honest feedback on this book as I hatched this idea, put words onto paper, removed and rewrote many of those words and added more and finally came up with this finished product.

To Stacia for showing amazing courage and setting a terrific example of how one deals with and thrives through cancer. While your age has not yet hit double digits, your maturity and wisdom far exceeds that of people much older than you.

To Lori, Mike, Bryce and Stacia: thank you for opening your home up to me as I recovered from my cancer surgery. Also to Mike, Bryce and Stacia: I appreciate you "loaning" Lori to me so that she could serve as Captain of my Boundary Buddies.

To Thom Hollis for his usual amazing job of cover design. His daughter Hannah added her creative touches to the cover design as well and her efforts are much appreciated.

To my friends and family who have helped me through the journey from diagnosis to New Normal. Listing you all by name is not feasible but know that you will always be in my heart.

To Jesus Christ, my Lord and Savior who is the constant foundation and focus of my life. I am nothing without Him.

MY CRAZY THYROID GLAND

Bob Seger was onto something when he sang "I feel like a number". According to the American Cancer Society in 2011, an estimated 37,000 women in the United States were diagnosed with thyroid cancer. On September 9, 2011, I became one of THOSE numbers of women. The reality is that such statistics become an entirely different story when you become one of those numbers.

This book is about my "entirely different story". In fact, every cancer patient's story is entirely different and as unique as their disease. Some will tell their stories as well while still others sadly did not live to share their experiences. While my story deals with thyroid cancer, some very universal themes exist across the broad spectrum of cancers. Whether a person's cancer is quite treatable, quickly terminal or somewhere in between, the word "cancer" has an impact that hits like a ton of bricks to the patient whose world has suddenly been turned upside down.

But let me begin by setting the stage of my life prior to the point cancer entered. I was born and raised in Idaho Falls, Idaho, a town located in the southeastern portion of the state. Idaho is shaped like a gun and Idaho Falls is in the handle. The main economic support of Idaho Falls is the nuclear industry via the Idaho National Engineering Laboratory (INEL) which is located near Arco, Idaho. Locals refer to the INEL as "The Site".

My parents met at The Site where Dad worked as an engineer and Mom as a secretary. They married and had six children, three boys and three girls. I am the fourth of the six and the youngest girl. Through words and action, Mom and Dad encouraged education and community involvement.

I grew up in a converted farmhouse sitting on just over an acre of land on the east side of Idaho Falls. The yard was filled with trees and gardens of all sizes and types. I learned many athletic skills playing softball and football in the front yard. My mom grew beautiful roses and iris and the trees were excellent places to curl up with a good book on a lazy day. However, life has not been all roses as I will share throughout this book.

Summer afternoons were often spent at combination BBQs and softball games at the family farm on the west side of town. Each July 4th, my mom would make homemade scones and a crowd of people would watch the parade go by our house. After the parade, we would have a snowball fight using the 30 gallon garbage sack of snow which had been sitting in our freezer since the winter months.

I lived in Idaho Falls through high school and then went to Moscow, Idaho to study computer science at the University of Idaho (UI) in the early 1980s. After I served as UI student body president, I dropped out to figure out what I wanted to do with my life. I returned to Idaho Falls and then moved to Boise, Idaho in 1988, and have lived here since then. In the mid 1990s, I went back to college and completed a degree in psychology with a minor in communication at Boise State University (BSU). Then, I did graduate work in communication at BSU and taught there for ten years. After experiencing a number of different jobs, I landed in my dream career of writing and publishing books. I will fill in more of the gaps in my life throughout this book.

Speaking of which...when I decided to write this book, I thought about the catchy opening I would have particularly about the moment I found out I had cancer. Well, there's no catchy way to describe what it's like to hit a brick wall. So rather than sugar coat it, let me take you to THE MOMENT!

Actually, there was not just one MOMENT but rather two moments: one moment was when I figured out I had cancer and one when I found out I had cancer. In terms of the first moment, as with so many other major events in one's life, I remember exactly where and what I was doing when I got the first phone call.

Like many folks, I am not the most coherent when the phone wakes me regardless of whether I am in a deep sleep or squeezing in an afternoon catnap as I was that day. I had taken my two Shih-Tzus, Mickey and Moose, into the backyard so they could run around and make sure the yard was properly defended against squirrels, insects, leaves and anything else that might threaten our collective safety. Although the heat was typical of an Idaho September late afternoon, I decided to nap on the swinging chair. I was in the midst of getting my company's latest book to publication and was particularly tired. The release party was in a month and I was dealing with 50 authors whose works were included in the book. I drifted off to sleep as the rhythm of the swing relaxed me.

I woke up when the phone rang and became coherent partway into the conversation. The call was from my internist's office to let me know that my thyroid blood test result had come back a bit off and the physician, Dr. Nona, wanted me to have a thyroid scan to make sure everything was OK. I stopped and let the words sink in as I was sure this was a case of déjà vu all over again.

"That can't be" I responded. "I had a call yesterday from your office telling me that my blood work was OK."

"That was a different blood test" replied the nurse. "Because of your family history, the doctor ordered another test just on your thyroid. She did not like the results and wants you to have a thyroid scan. You will get a call to have that scan scheduled in the next week or so. Once the doctor has a chance to review those results, we'll be back in touch. Do you have any questions?"

"Questions?" I thought to myself. Of course I have questions, but I could not think of a single one at that point. "No, I do not have any questions," I replied. I thanked her for calling me and hung up.

I was in shock. What was my crazy thyroid gland up to? If the nurse had mentioned just about any other part of my body, the idea of a scan would not have had nearly the impact. However, the words "thyroid" and "family history" were a different story as two other members of my immediate family had had thyroid cancer. At that moment, I knew that I was headed down the same road and that I had thyroid cancer, but there were more steps to come before I received the definitive word from my doctor.

The amazing part to me was that I had no symptoms. I had felt good and gone in for my annual physical. Dr. Nona, whom I had been going to for about 15 years, had palpitated my thyroid and not felt anything. Because of my family history, she decided to do an extra blood test; a fact I had forgotten until just a few minutes before when I had received the test results from her office.

I sat on the swing lost in thought as I tried to figure out what my next steps should be. I knew that I needed two things at this point: prayer and information.

In 1988, I accepted Jesus Christ as my Lord and Savior in what has been the most important decision I have made in my life. Having that core foundation has brought me through crises that would have been disastrous if I had tried to handle them on my own. Do not get me wrong; I still believed that at times God was too busy with other situations so in order to help out, I would rely on myself and not seek His guidance (refer back to that disastrous comment).

However, I was fortunate at the point of my cancer diagnosis that I was much better about taking things to God and not trying to solve them myself. The same holds true today and is getting even more frequent as I know that the Lord has a much better handle on "the bigger picture" than I could ever hope to see, let alone comprehend.

For much of my Christian walk, I have been guilty of seeing God as a prayer vending machine. I tell Him what I want (not necessarily need) and He will give it to me. How rude is that? I have no children that I am aware of, but if I did have a child and all he or she did was ask for stuff, I would be beyond annoyed. Yet the Lord does not get annoyed with me and continually waits for me to figure out that He is NOT a prayer vending machine.

I say continually because having Jesus Christ as my Lord and Savior is both a process and an event but is actually in reverse order. For example, getting a college degree is an event, but the process is just as important. The two times I went to college were very different as I was 17 when I entered the University of Idaho and 32 as I began my student career at Boise State University. Although I did not get a degree at UI and did at BSU, both processes taught me a great deal about myself. Yet in my Christian walk, the event of accepting Jesus Christ as my Lord and Savior came first and the process of living a life worthy of Him followed. If I waited until I had my life in order to come to the Lord, I still would not have a personal relationship with Him. Thankfully, I simply had to confess my sins and to recognize Jesus Christ as Lord and Savior and the process began.

For me, that process continues to include a growing reliance on prayer but with a minimalistic vending machine approach. Instead, I approach my prayer time with the Lord as an opportunity to hold a conversation and to get insights. This method involves spending more time listening than talking. I wholeheartedly agree with the belief that we have two ears and one mouth and they should be used proportionally.

As somebody who has a bent toward science and such, I also look to the research as to the effects of prayer. Arguments go back and forth as to the benefits of prayer and such debates will continue. However what I see is that prayer has physical and psychological benefits regardless of whether the prayer is answered. Simply put, people feel better when they pray. Another interesting fact is that according to Dr. Larry Dossey "In 1993, only three U.S. medical schools had courses devoted to exploring the role of religious practice and prayer in health; currently, nearly 80 medical schools have instituted such courses."

Regardless, I have seen what praying does in my life and in the life of others. With my crazy gland now containing cancer, I was going to do some praying myself and ask others to do the same. But I knew that part of that process meant gathering more information as I had a bunch of questions and knew others would too.

Oh and how much information is available! Simply put, we live in an Information Age on steroids. Between an Internet bigger than we can comprehend, more books than we could ever read and more radio, television and media sources than we could ever access, we are FLOODED with information.

For example, watch an old television news broadcast and compare it to one of today. I grew up watching Chet Huntley, David Brinkley and Walter Cronkite. They would read the news from sheets of paper while some information may appear in a small screen next to their heads. Such information would include a map of where the event was occurring or perhaps some statistics. The newscaster would also introduce a story to be reported by a journalist in the field or who was sitting at the same desk. The key was one story at a time with one piece of information at a time. Furthermore, news was reported from the national media one time per night while the local stations would do two broadcasts a night: one usually after the national newscast and then one after prime time television ended for the evening.

Fast forward ahead to newscasts today. While in the Huntley/Brinkley/Cronkite days, information was reported one piece at a time at a slower pace, today's newscasts are much different. In addition to the information that is shared on the story being reported, the viewer can keep up on stock prices, sports scores and other news items by watching the streaming tickers across the bottom of the screen. Even the pieces of paper from which the news are reported have been replaced by Teleprompters to give the subtle message that news is fresh and not old.

In addition, news reporting is no longer limited to a few times per day but rather can be accessed 24 hours a day on multiple channels (let alone via the Internet). We are even reminded how busy the news people are by the images of folks scurrying around behind the on-air person. There is so much to report that they have to stay constantly busy to capture all of the "important stories".

However, the information can be too much. During 9/11, I remember friends of mine sharing that their young children came to them and asked if the parents would turn off the televisions. The combination of the emotional shock of the events and our "need to know" produced information overload as our collective society tried to search for answers in the details of the day.

With any information we receive, we have two options: discard it or retain it. The information that we discard either consciously or subconsciously is like water off a duck's back. On the other hand, the information we retain becomes knowledge.

Filtering through what to discard and what to retain can be quite a challenge so discernment is important. I look for collaborating sources to the information and rarely rely on simply one resource to determine the validity of what I have read, heard, seen or otherwise consumed. This practice became even more important as I was dealing with the repercussions of my crazy thyroid gland. As I will share more throughout this book, I used some more specific techniques to deal with all of the information I had to consume along my cancer journey.

Speaking of information consumed, let me explain the difference between the two blood tests I had regarding my thyroid. One test was to measure my TSH or Thyroid Stimulating Hormone. That number indicates normal, hypothyroidism or hyperthyroidism. Normal speaks for itself while hypothyroidism means the thyroid is operating too slowly and hyperthyroidism means that crazy gland is working too fast. The normal range is subject for debate so I suggest reading Mary Shomon's book "Living Well with Hypothyroidism". She does an excellent job of demystifying the thyroid and the various illnesses associated with that crazy gland.

While my TSH level did not raise concern, the result of the other thyroid blood test did catch Dr.

Nona's attention. That test is for Tg or Thyroglobulin which can be a tumor marker for papillary or follicular thyroid cancer. My level was 23 which set off bells and whistles in Dr. Nona's head and resulted in her sending me for a thyroid scan. The Tg test is one that getting a 0 on is the goal!

As promised, the next week I had a phone call setting up the scan. The purpose of the scan was to determine if a tumor or tumors were visible on my thyroid. I found myself plunging into a world I had not visited in decades. I had enjoyed very good health for many years and had not had surgery in over 30 years. I had my routine physicals over the years and other than a concussion about five years prior, I had not been in a hospital except to visit other people who were patients. Furthermore, I had not carried health insurance for many years until a couple of months prior to the start of my cancer journey.

When I arrived at the facility to have the scan of my thyroid, I began what would become a routine over the weeks and months to come: fill out paperwork, produce insurance cards, recite the Pledge of Allegiance, sign forms, and provide medical history and medicines taken. The scan took almost no time compared to what was involved in paperwork, histories, insurance, etc. Oh and yes, I was kidding about that reciting the Pledge of Allegiance part.

The young woman who performed the scan was very polite and professional and we chatted as she did her work. Now I had been through enough of these kinds of procedures as I accompanied my parents to their medical appointments to know the answer to the question I was about to ask, but I figured it could not hurt to try:

"So how does it look?" I asked the technician. I knew she would not be able to tell me, but I was looking for what she did not say. As I mentioned earlier, I taught communication at Boise State University and continued to present and to consult on the topic after I left BSU in 2007. One point I remember and continue to emphasize is that up to 90% of any given communication is nonverbal. In other words, we say more with how we say something than what we say.

"You'll have to wait and talk with the radiologist," she replied politely. The fact that she would not look me in the eye indicated to me that the news was probably bad. I say "probably" because nonverbal communication is NOT an exact science. For example, if somebody folds their arms that does not necessarily mean they are mad; in fact, they could be cold or contemplating something. However, in past situations when helping others who were undergoing medical procedures, I could often get some sort of response from a technician if the news was good. So, I was not thinking good news about my thyroid was in my future.

And so the saga continued: a couple of days later, Dr. Nona's office called to say they were referring me to an endocrinologist who would recommend how to proceed. Doctors do not usually just refer people to specialists for the fun of it so I knew that all was not hunky-dory in Jane's Thyroid Land. Within several days, the call came from the endocrinologist's office and my quickly scheduled appointment was at hand.

At this point, I thanked God for the experience I had gained through walking along with my parents through their health problems as they aged. Paul, one of my brothers, and I took turns accompanying Mom and Dad to their appointments as our schedules worked out. Paul (AKA P.D.) lived in Idaho Falls near Mom and Dad but traveled a lot for his work. I lived four hours away from Idaho Falls in Boise and would head to my native land as needed to help out. P.D. and I would coordinate with Mom and Dad about which appointments they wanted somebody to go to with them and then make arrangements according to our work schedules.

Through those appointments, I learned about listening to what the health care professionals were saying and what they were not saying. I respect the patient by letting them take the lead and ask questions as appropriate. I take notes and try to write as legibly as possible as sometimes the speed of speech was faster than that of my hand.

Another important lesson I learned was how to ask for clarification when I sensed inconsistency, particularly when the verbal communication collided with the nonverbal communication. I believe that the number one rule of improved communication is "When in doubt, ask". The word "doubt" means to be of double mind as shown by the "doub" portion. So if I am of double mind about a particular subject, I ask. In a number of cases, asking is a delicate skill to be practiced and to be honed as some doctors do not like their assessments questioned. Oh well, it's not their health.

The other experience I was thankful for was the organized approach my dad, a chemical and nuclear engineer, took to managing his health care. He created two significant computer documents I used as models for my own journey. The first file summarized the medicines he was taking including dosage, frequency and the doctor who prescribed them. Whenever a prescription was changed, Dad would fax the updated table to all of his doctors.

The other document summarized our family medical history on both Mom and Dad's sides of the family. Both Mom and Dad were very open about the illnesses, conditions and other medical information they knew of in their respective families. Gathering the information for Mom's side was relatively easy (pun intended). Mom and her five brothers, their wives and families lived pretty much in the Idaho Falls area. In addition, Grandma Hansen (AKA Mom's Mom) was a regular part of our lives as she stayed near the family farm after Grandpa Hansen died when Mom was 18. The sources were present so getting a family medical history for the Hansen side of the family was easier.

The same could not be said for Dad's side of the family as he did not know most of his relatives. A native of Vienna, Austria, Dad was an only child whose mother died when he was six weeks old and whose father died when he was about seven. The grandparents who raised him sent him to live in America when Dad was eleven years old and were subsequently murdered at Auschwitz. Dad filled in his medical history with what he knew about his family through his young memory and conversations he had with his few surviving cousins.

So armed with what I had learned from Mom and Dad, I created the medical history and medicines taking documents and prepared my list of questions for meeting with the endocrinologist. Now I will admit that I did not go into this appointment with the best of attitudes and the reason was not the cancer question but rather had to do with my doctor experiences accompanying Mom, Dad and others.

In my opinion, doctors fall into one of four categories: (1) good doctoring skills with good communication skills, (2) good doctoring with lousy communication skills, (3) lousy doctoring with good communication skills and (4) lousy doctoring with lousy communication skills. I believe that lousy communication skills can be overcome with good questioning and information gathering, but lousy doctoring skills requires a change in physicians.

That said, I would take a doctor who falls into one of the first two categories over a physician who falls into one of the latter two categories. In fact, these four categories are listed in order of my preference. Unfortunately in assisting others, I interacted with several doctors who fell into categories (3) and (4). Consequently, I expected the same results when I started seeing more doctors in my cancer journey.

Fortunately, I was pleasantly surprised when I met the endocrinologist, Dr. Richard Christensen. From the time he shook my hand when we met, Dr. Christensen was knowledgeable and friendly and definitely fell into category (1). That made the news he was about to give me a bit easier to swallow (yes the pun was intended as I deliberately made a joke about swallowing in relation to my thyroid).

He explained that the thyroid looks like two teaspoons side-by-side. The scan showed two small growths on the top of my thyroid: one on the left side and one on the right. Some other tiny growths peppered the bottom half of the thyroid, but they were too small to be biopsied. We had a very candid discussion about how comfortable I would be with the idea of these tumors which may or may not be cancerous hanging out in my throat.

As Dr. Christensen and I were having this discussion, I had two major thoughts running through my head. One was the first time I met Dr. Brenda Williams, who became my gynecologist. Brenda was the keynote speaker at the Survivors Dinner for the Susan G. Komen Breast Cancer Foundation Boise Race for the Cure, an organization which I helped with on marketing and publicity.

As a breast cancer survivor, Brenda spoke of the 500 pound gorilla she lived with every day; that is the knowledge that the cancer could possibly come back. She commented that she was learning to live with the gorilla because she was down to doing self-breast exams only once or twice a day. Brenda's quick wit was wonderful and I remember her fondly. Unfortunately, the gorilla came to stay permanently several years later as Brenda had another cancer battle, but this one she lost. She died in 2009 at the age of 55.

The other major thought that was bouncing around my brain as Dr. Christensen and I discussed my health was my belief about lymph nodes: they are the cancer highway. Whenever I heard of some-body having cancer, one of my main concerns was "Did the disease spread to the lymph nodes?" If that was the case, the cancer could go anywhere because lymph nodes are all over the body. Once the disease hits the lymphatic system, fighting the cancer can be more difficult. Well, I am no Marcus Welby but I knew from my anatomy and physiology classes in college that the thyroid has lymph nodes on either side of it. Cancer does not ask permission to invade our bodies let alone jump into the lymph nodes so why give it the opportunity? Add into the equation my family history of thyroid cancer and I did not need any more discussion. I would have the biopsy to get the cancer question answered.

Dr. Christensen explained that he would do a needle biopsy of the two larger tumors on either side of the top of the thyroid gland. My peppered pals across the bottom half of my crazy gland would be too small to get enough needle biopsy tissue samples for testing. However, he would take several samples of each of the two larger tumors to determine if they were malignant or benign. When he stood up, I ex-pected Dr. Christensen to say that he would go check to see when the biopsy could be scheduled. "Let me go move my next appointment and we'll do the biop-sy right now," he said and then left the room.

I was stunned! I expected to get the medical runaround and have to come back another day and not anytime soon. Instead within a few minutes, Dr. Christensen and his nurse were prepping me and numbing the area of my neck where the needle biop-sy would be done. They explained that I would feel some pressure as the needle was inserted and that some bruising would occur around the sites where the needle entered and exited my neck. Soon, the biopsy was over and the samples on their way to the lab where they would be tested and some major next steps in my life would be determined. The nurse said they would have results a couple of days later and would call me.

For now though, I had to live my life as I knew it. For me, that meant continuing to prepare for the book release party which was now just a couple of weeks away. I had interviews to prepare for as well as dealing with dozens of excited authors who were looking forward to the release of the book. Also, I had the well-wishers who wanted to know what was happening with my thyroid. I developed a "no news is good news" policy and said I would let them know when I knew more and I kept living life.

That Friday, September 9, 2011, living life meant taking my cat Theolonius to the vet. I have three cats and two dogs, four of whom are over ten years of age and thus are geriatric in my book. Having elderly felines and canines means that I spend a lot of time at my veterinarians' office. I spend so much time there that they greet me with "Jane" with the same familiarity with which Norm was welcomed on Cheers.

Theolonius looks like a black panther version of a domestic cat. At 16 pounds, he could have passed for a small panther but has a very sweet disposition. Theolonius was likely not properly weaned from his mother because he likes sitting in the crook of my arm and kneading my bicep with his paws.

Theolonius seems to be trying to get milk out of my elbow and in ten years of trying, he has yet to succeed.

Well, that particular day, my beautiful black cat had his turn to visit the veterinarian. I do not remember the ailment, but I do know it was something that necessitated not waiting until the next week. Theolonius slept on the passenger seat while I drove because he did not feel like driving.

As a general rule, I do not talk on my phone while I am driving, so when the automated voice announced that the call was from Dr. Christensen's office, I pulled into a parking lot to answer my phone. At this point, because the car was stopped and hearing a voice he did not know, Theolonius woke up and decided to start prowling around the car including over my shoulder, across my lap and on my head. Not easy to have a serious phone conversation when a 16 pound cat is using me as a climbing toy. Thankfully, he was not employing me as a scratching post.

The woman on the other end of the phone wanted to know if I could come in that afternoon to talk about my biopsy results. That request along with the urgency in her voice and the fact that it was a Friday afternoon told me that the news was not good. If the tests had shown no cancer, she could let me know that news and wish me a pleasant weekend with the knowledge that she had removed a huge weight from my life.

Instead, she wanted to see me in person as she clearly and correctly did not want to deliver the bombshell over the phone. After all, I would have questions and emotional reactions that should be dealt with and not left to stew over a weekend (particularly with the Internet at my disposal which would lead to more questions than answers). Besides, she was confirming what I had already figured out: I had thyroid cancer. I also had a cat that needed to go to the vet right then and there. Theolonius' health would be better in a matter of hours after he was examined and appropriately medicated by the vet. I was in for a much longer haul.

So, I explained that today would not work as I was taking my cat to the veterinarian, but that I was available on Monday. However, I wanted her to know that I understood the seriousness of the situation; that is, I knew what she was not saying: I had thyroid cancer. "I'm OK with waiting until meeting with the doctor on Monday," I replied. "My dad had thyroid cancer and I have a pretty good knowledge of the disease."

Clearly relieved, she explained that Dr. Christensen would not be in on Monday, but that I could meet with his physician's assistant. I explained that would be fine with me and thanked her for the phone call.

I found out what I had figured out and the journey had begun...

YOU PUT MUSTARD ON MY CHEESEBURGER! DON'T YOU KNOW I HAVE CANCER?

The following Monday, I went into to Dr. Christensen's office to meet with his physician's assistant. She explained that I had papillary thyroid cancer as the results showed that one of the two tumors on the top of my thyroid was malignant and that the other tumor was suspicious. Whether the second tumor was cancerous would not be confirmed or denied until the tests were done when the tumor was removed. Whether my peppered pals across the bottom of my thyroid were malignant or benign would be determined when they were taken out during surgery.

So the next step would be surgery, but in the meantime, I went into information gathering mode. I had some background knowledge about thyroid cancer having walked along with Dad through his illness. He had given me various articles to read and answered my questions about his cancer. Dad had had his entire thyroid removed and that was followed up with RAI or Radioactive Iodine. When Dad underwent RAI, he spent a few days in the basement away from Mom and other people and creatures as to not expose them. Being the thorough people they were, Mom and Dad had made up a list of questions for the doctor about what to do with dishes Dad used, clothes he wore and other items he touched while he had the RAI. I am so thankful that my parents were such detail-oriented people as shown through Dad's cancer treatment. I used that approach and foundation of knowledge to help me as I began gathering information on my thyroid cancer.

As I said at the start of this book, each person's cancer story is different and so were the journeys of my dad and me. First of all, over 13 years passed between Dad's diagnosis in the spring of 1998 and mine in the fall of 2011 so diagnosis and treatment had changed. In addition, Dad's cancer had spread beyond his thyroid and mine appeared to be contained to my crazy gland. That last fact meant that I would likely not be having RAI but that would not be known for certain until after my surgery.

At this point, like many others in my life, my natural curiosity bode me well. When I was a child, my parents gave me a series of three books titled "Tell Me Why" and those volumes are still on my shelf over 40 years later. Some of the information in those books is still correct while other data is outdated. However, the premise of the book still exists and as I pointed out earlier: when of double mind, that is "in doubt", ask. So, I started reviewing what I knew and began asking as much as I could before I met with the surgeon.

I knew enough about papillary thyroid cancer to know that it was not fast growing and that time was on my side. I did not have to make decisions from a point of panic but had the benefit of having some time to research and to process before making decisions. I was referred to Dr. Todd Rudstad, a surgeon with a great deal of experience in treating thyroid cancer. That appointment would come, but for now I had life to live in addition to planning what to do about my new friend thyroid cancer.

For me, life meant continuing the work on the release of my latest book at that time: "An Eclectic Collage Volume 2: Relationships of Life". When I say "my book", I mean that the work was published by my company, but the book itself had 50 women authors which made for all sorts of logistical challenges on my part. However, like making laws and sausage, the process was ugly at times but turned out well in the end.

So a few weeks after my cancer diagnosis, I had the privilege of doing a book signing in Crouch, a small town tucked away about an hour north of Boise. Idaho has become a place where people from other states come to retire so tiny towns are popping up all over the place. The natives and the newbies strike a comfortable balance of existence as they realize we all pretty much came from someplace else.

Crouch is a nice place and I was particularly excited because I was going to see my friend, Judy, who doubles as the mother of my friend Lori. Judy was not going to be able to stay for the book signing as she had a previous commitment, but we still were going to be able to connect for a few minutes before she had to leave.

In her usual thoughtful way, Judy had a present for me: a Moxie Java coffee shop gift card, coffee cup and a magnetic cross with the word "JOURNEY" across it and Jeremiah 29:11 written on it as well: "For I know the plans I have for you says the Lord. They are plans for good and not for disaster, to give you a future and a hope." I commented that the same verse had been the theme of a women's church retreat I had attended a couple of years ago.

As I said thanks and gave Judy a hug, she said that I should come back to Crouch sometime because "you need to meet Janet. She's an author too and has written books about having breast cancer." I smiled and said that Lori had told me that "Mom has an author she wants you to meet."

After Judy left, I went into the bookstore to set up for the signing and wait for the arrival of Carolyn, one of the co-authors of the book we were in Crouch to promote. As I settled in, I looked up to see one of the event organizers walking in with another woman. She began to say that this woman was also an author and had written about having breast cancer. Well, Crouch is not that big and so I took a chance and said: "You must be Janet. Judy has told me a lot about you and suggested we meet." Indeed, I had met Janet.

The two of us began talking about our writing and publishing history and I discovered how accomplished she is as a writer. Janet had books published by "big dogs" like Simon and Schuster and Lifeway. However, Janet was very humble about her experiences which made a much better impression on me than if she had dropped big names like lead weights.

Then Janet shared that she had just gone through her third battle with breast cancer. I told her that I had been recently diagnosed with thyroid cancer. We chatted back and forth, but our focus quickly turned to the folks who had come to the event.

Soon a group of about six or seven women gathered and the suggestion was made that we read from the Eclectic Collage Volume 2 book. I began by reading a couple of short stories related to various relationships and then Carolyn read her essay about finding and meeting her birth mother. Tears were being shed all over the room and I found myself welling up too because I had been more emotional than usual.

For the first few weeks since I found out I had thyroid cancer, I operated in the "head knowledge" portion of facing the disease. I knew that I had an excellent likelihood of beating this illness and was thankful that I had "cancer" and not "CANCER" (that is a type that was more serious and difficult to treat).

However, I knew the reality as shared with me by an old friend facing off against a totally different illness. She began dealing with her alcoholism telling me that she was not like other alcoholics and that failed miserably. Only when she realized that she was no different was she able to begin her real recovery. She was dead on and her now two years of sobriety shows it.

Well, I realized that I AM like others who have or have had cancer. In other words, my head told my heart I have cancer and thus needed to face the emotional reality of the disease. For somebody like me who is used to getting through projects by making and executing to-do lists and setting aside time to get the job done, this realization threw me for a loop.

However, as I was reminded as I prayed, I could not schedule my way through emotions but rather had to let them happen as they do. This point was emphasized when I opened up Sarah Young's

"Jesus Calling", a book of daily devotions given to me by Lori. That day's entry said "Do not rush the process". OK, God...point made.

All of this was whirling around me throughout the book signing. As I was autographing books for a woman named Diane, she told me that she had had breast cancer twice. When Janet came back our way, I told her of Diane's victories and they began to share stories while I signed books.

Then Janet asked me about what my treatment was going to be. I told her and Diane that I would be meeting with the surgeon the next week, but I thought I was facing having my thyroid removed and then possibly three days of at-home radiation. Then I switched gears and told them about hitting the emotional wall that past weekend.

I was sitting in a chair and Janet and Diane were standing next to me and I will always remember the looks on their faces. These sisters in survival, who had beaten cancer five times between the two of them, had a combination of empathy and understanding in their eyes that resembled a knowing peace. They had been there and knew exactly what I was talking about.

Then I relayed to them my feelings of anger about my cancer. I told them the night before I had stopped for a hamburger on my way to a Bible study. I rarely eat fast food anymore, but I was particularly hungry so a hamburger and fries sounded very good. I am a "plain Jane" eater as I did not care much for condiments and ordered my usual cheeseburger with lettuce, onion and tomato only.

I drove out of the Wendy's parking lot and onto the freeway. As I bit into the hamburger, I discovered that they had put the dreaded and disgusting condiment known as mustard on my cheeseburger. Even though I knew it would make me late, I took the next exit and doubled back to get my cheeseburger made correctly. I calmly explained what had happened and a new cheeseburger was cooked to order. What I really wanted to do was scream "You put mustard on my cheeseburger. Don't you know I have cancer!!!?"

As I told Janet and Diane this story, they nodded and had the same compassionate looks on their faces. Janet commented that I sounded like I was grieving and said she wanted to give me a copy of her book which discussed stages of grieving cancer. Even though our cancer types were different, Janet thought I would benefit from reading her book (which is titled "Dear God, They Say It's Cancer").

I gave both Janet and Diane one of my business cards and asked them to stay in touch. They each gave me a hug when they left; two hours before we were total strangers and yet we now shared a common bond. As I prepared for the event that night, I was planning to sign books and to meet readers. However, in His Jeremiah 29:11 way, God had other plans for me in Crouch: He wanted to comfort my soul. He knew that what I REALLY needed was to meet Janet and Diane and, as usual, He was correct.

Now that my head and heart were both in the game, my real cancer journey had begun.

MY CANCER PLATE

I am likely in the minority with this statement, but I really enjoyed elementary, junior high and high schools. School did a lot to fan the flame of my love of learning. In addition, I met all kinds of terrific people in the forms of classmates and teachers. Over the years, I have maintained contact with many of them and enjoy sharing old stories as well as catching up on what's new in life. The past is a great place to visit, but my best days are ahead of and not behind me.

Reconnecting with friends from those various stages of my life is a pleasure when we do not get caught in the past. School was the place we met and that shared past gives us common memories. But life goes on and those childhood friendships that are the strongest are when we support and encourage one another through the realness of adulthood.

I reconnected with two such childhood friends a few years ago after my 30-year high school class reunion. Julie, Shelly, Leila and I had attended O.E. Bell Junior High together in the mid-1970s before we parted ways. The three of them went to Idaho Falls High School (IFHS) while I went across town to Skyline High School. Julie and I stayed in touch as we played recreational softball together in high school and then both attended the University of Idaho. Over the years, Julie and I have remained good friends.

On the other hand, Shelly and Leila maintained contact as they both attended Idaho State University where Shelly studied pharmacy and Leila focused on accounting. Both of them had married and each had two boys. Except for running into Shelly at a drugstore where she worked in the 1990s, I had not seen either she or Leila for over 35 years even though we all lived in the Boise area. However the year 2010 marked our respective 30 year high school reunions so reminiscing was in the air. Julie, Shelly and Leila had their IFHS class reunion several weeks before mine for Skyline. As the three of them reconnected, they talked about hooking up with me and Julie took the bull by the horns. In the fall of 2010, Julie e-mailed to set up a lunch with the four of us.

Syncing up our schedules proved to be a bit of a challenge, but we finally found a time to have lunch on a beautiful fall day in downtown Boise. We caught up on old classmates we had seen at our respective reunions and laughed about our junior high days. Leila claimed that I was the reason she made it through geometry while I think she helped me as much as I helped her. Julie and I talked about being Mathletes together and going to various competitions.

Speaking of competition, Julie, Shelly and I reminisced about playing ninth grade basketball together. Shelly was the kind of player under the basket that I was glad was on my team and not somebody I had to face. Julie used her height to her advantage as she had a terrific shot. I subbed in as guard and forward and enjoyed the camaraderie of the team sport (which is a very nice way of saying that I was not that good of a player).

As the lunch wound down, we planned on getting back together despite our busy schedules.

However with the friendships reconnected, Shelly and Leila joined Julie in being an important part of my thyroid cancer journey.

As I have mentioned before, I have been blessed with good health throughout the years. I had surgery in 1980 but did not stay again in a hospital until my cancer surgery. My medicine needs had been primarily non-prescription as I took vitamins and other supplements. I was reminded of this fact when just a month before my cancer diagnosis, one of my cats bit me and the wound became infected. The doctor at the urgent care facility prescribed an antibiotic and I had to figure out where to get the prescription filled as I had not had such a need in about 10 years.

Enter Shelly, my friend, and soon to be my pharmacist. As she was not working the day I needed the antibiotic and I did not know the location of her pharmacy, I had the prescription filled by another drugstore. I regretted that decision as that pharmacist neglected to tell me that this antibiotic was very powerful and would kill good bacteria as well. I had to deal with the "consequences" of that antibiotic which is a very nice way of saying that I had to stick close to the bathroom. So, I called Shelly who told me that the solution to my problem was to eat a yogurt every day to replenish my good antibiotic supply. I thanked her for the advice, not knowing that in just a few weeks she would be offering more where that came from.

Once I was diagnosed with thyroid cancer, I asked Shelly if we could have coffee so I could pick her brain about what I might be facing. As a pharmacist, Shelly saw firsthand the various treatment methods that were used to deal with thyroid issues. I had already begun hearing different pieces of information from people as to the main thyroid replacement drugs (Synthroid, Levothyroxine which is generic Synthroid, and pig thyroid). As was to become customary for me through my cancer journey, I developed a list of questions to ask; this time, the questions were for Shelly. The piece of our conversation that has stuck with me the longest did not come from Shelly, my pharmacist but rather from Shelly, my friend.

One of the nicest things anybody ever said to me was "Jane, you radiate realness". I strive to be genuine and do not have much use for phony. Ephesians 4:15 exhorts us to speak the truth in love to one another and that skill is something that is consistent across my closest friends. I say "skill" because speaking the truth in love takes practice and involves knowing when to speak the truth and when to keep your mouth shut. Simply because something is true does not mean that it needs to be said at that very moment. Those who are good at speaking the truth in love are perceptive as when doing so can be hurtful and when it can be helpful.

In Shelly's case, the truth she spoke to me in love was quite timely and thus very helpful. As we sat in the coffee shop sipping our respective beverages, Shelly looked at me with that same determined look I had seen many times on the basketball court when she was grabbing a rebound or breaking out of a double-team under the basket. She very quietly, forcefully and lovingly said, "You need to put Jane first here."

I did not reply but rather let her words sink in to my mind, heart and soul. As I processed them, I knew that Shelly was right. I was better at pouring myself out for others than I was keeping my own tanks filled. In order to recover from my cancer, I was going to have to take better care of myself and let others help me as well. I have always been good at asking for help when I need it but admittedly needed work on the self-care front. I tucked that one away for further and continual processing.

Shelly provided me with further sage advice on preparing for surgery and recovery as well as little personal details I had not further considered. Both being animal lovers, Shelly and I had shared many stories about our respective menageries. She walked me through all of the arrangements I had made for the animals to ensure that I had covered all of the bases. Her attention to doggy and kitty detail was much appreciated as my brain was otherwise focused on my cancer.

On the other hand, Leila and my first conversation after my cancer diagnosis took a different direction. Admittedly, I did not know Leila as well because junior high school was more Raging Hormone Land than Deep Friendshipville. Leila and I had Geometry and other classes together and ate lunch together at times but did not hang out a great deal outside of school. Yet as we drank coffee that Saturday morning in my new world where cancer lived, Leila made an analogy which became a cornerstone of explaining relationships as part of my cancer journey.

"Jane, it's like you have this cancer plate," Leila began as she formed her thumbs and forefingers into the shape of a plate. Putting her hand into a fist, she said, "And your cancer is small because it's very treatable and beatable. But the whole rest of the plate is filled with people trying to work through THEIR issues using YOUR cancer."

As with Shelly's self-care revelation, I sat in silence as I soaked in Leila's cancer plate analogy. She was right on the mark! In just the week since my diagnosis, I already saw people bringing their "stuff" to my cancer journey which is a very nice way of saying their issues came flying out of hiding.

Of course, each of us has issues which cloud our perceptions, but when somebody is facing a major illness or other challenge, she or he and their needs should come first. If you have a need to make their struggle about you, perhaps you need to re-examine your motives and step back from the situation. Particularly during the initial days of my cancer diagnosis, the last thing I needed was somebody trying to make my illness about them. For example, friends who had had cancer insisted I see their doctors even though thyroid cancer was out of their areas of expertise. Other friends would tell me what I HAD to do without ever asking how I was doing. With her "Cancer Plate" analogy, Leila had put a clear visual to what I was feeling as I was reeling from my cancer diagnosis.

In the days after Leila's amazing insight, I realized a change to the analogy was in order. I needed to examine my boundaries and adjust them to my "New Normal" of having cancer. However, I knew that I could not do this boundary building and tweaking on my own but was going to need some help. I needed good boundaries between me and all of the well-meaning people who were trying to work through their issues using my cancer. I envisioned myself and my cancer with a group of "Boundary Buddies" who would deal with these well-meaning folks for I did not have the strength or inclination to do so.

Over the next few weeks, a group of friends emerged who became my Boundary Buddies. They would each serve different roles at various points through my cancer journey. Also, each of my Boundary Buddies has the common characteristic of knowing when to dive in and when to back off. I knew that I needed somebody to lead the charge and did not even hesitate as to who she would be.

I have a natural fascination with the subject of friendships thanks in part to the fact that my last name means "friend" in German. The other foundation of the fascination comes from the reality that my friends have helped me through some of the most difficult times I have ever faced. However, through the course of my life, I have been blessed beyond belief with absolutely amazing friends! I am continually in awe of how the Lord brings people into, back through, or briefly a part of my life. I have deep meaningful friendships that range from one of 45 years which began at the age of four to ones that have existed for a fraction of that time. However, when I looked for the Captain of the Boundary Bud-

dies, I went to a friendship that was only a couple of
years old. I chose Lori.

CAPTAIN LORI OF THE BOUNDARY BUDDIES

Have you ever noticed that there is a one letter difference between "mother" and "smother"? Well, I had because I began living it once the word got out that I had thyroid cancer. Perhaps because some folks recognized that I had lost my own mother just two years before, well-meaning women wanted to fill that role. Another very plausible theory is that because I am single and have never been married (that I am aware of), I would need extra help as I apparently had not been able to manage the nearly 30 years I had been on my own. All jokes aside, the response was both quite touching and overwhelming. I heard from many people who wanted to know how I was doing, what they could do to help and other variations of good deeds.

My head was still spinning and I had no idea what I needed let alone how to go about dealing with the various inquiries, well-wishers, etc. I did not know what I did not know, but fortunately I had somebody who did and who was willing to help me in whatever ways possible: my friend Lori. Fortunately, she had experience in this cancer journey and was a bit further down that path.

God has an amazing way of putting very important people in our lives long before they serve the crucial role He has planned for them. In September 2009, I went to Cascade, Idaho to speak at a women's retreat for Foothills Christian Church of Boise. The topic of the retreat was about friendship which is near and dear to my heart as my first book was a

Bible study on women's friendships. I had spent a great deal of time working with the retreat planning committee so I was particularly invested in not getting in God's way as He spoke to the women who attended the retreat.

But I also knew that the Lord would be speaking a great deal to me as well on that particular weekend. Just three weeks before, my mom died as a result of a fall in her home. Mom's health had been declining for years and she never really recovered from a broken hip and leg she had sustained in 2005. So, I had had some time to prepare for Mom's death, but the event was a moving target as I had no idea when she would die.

Then the phone call came one Sunday in late August 2009 that Mom had fallen and I drove from Boise to Idaho Falls to see her in the hospital. Within 24 hours, she had suffered two grand mal seizures and the determination was that she was not a candidate for surgery. A few days later on her 78th birthday, Mom came home for the last time. She died that Saturday evening with one of my sisters and me at her side.

Mom's death brought the end to an important chapter in my life: I had lost both of my parents. Regardless of age, having your last parent die creates a feeling of being an orphan. I remember when my Grandma Hansen, died nearly 50 years after Grandpa Hansen's death. Mom and her five brothers were all in their 60s or 70s at the time with children, grandchildren and even great-grandchildren. Yet Mom and some of my uncles commented that Grandma's death made them feel like orphans.

That orphan feeling along with some other family health and related issues made for a very difficult time for me. My brother Paul (P.D.) had a benign brain tumor removed in November 2006, just four months after Dad had died. During the surgery, Paul suffered a stroke which left him with permanent disabilities. Since we were children, Paul and I had been very close. Although Paul is four years younger than me, we have been mistaken for twins as our mannerisms, features and voices are quite similar. Paul feigned horror when he was called a "male Jane" by one of our friends but both of us were flattered by the comparison. As adults, Paul and I had many dinners together in Boise when he traveled through on business.

The night of Mom's funeral, I found out that Paul's benign brain tumor had returned and he would be having more surgery. . This news was particularly devastating to me and I had a heavy heart when I returned to Boise to prepare for the retreat.

The ladies of Foothills Christian Church could not have been more wonderful to me through this process. When I arrived back to Boise, I had a lovely plant they had sent me extending their sympathies on Mom's death. They gave me the opportunity to withdraw as the retreat speaker and I prayed and contemplated whether I should take them up on their very kind offer. In the end, I knew that speaking would be healing for me as I do much of my processing by talking. I needed to share what Mom had meant to me.

I was very fortunate that my dear friend, Ellen, had long ago agreed to accompany me to the Foothills Women's Retreat. Getting our schedules in sync has always been a challenge so we make the most of the time we are able to have together. The idea that we would have uninterrupted driving time to and from Cascade as well as nuggets of conversation throughout the weekend was quite appealing to both of us as we could catch up on our lives. Ellen is the type of friend where we might have minimal face-to-face contact for weeks, but when we do get together, we pick up where we left off.

Ellen walked along with me through my Dad's death and helped me through that traumatic time. I had been in regular contact with her as Mom was dying and Paul was having surgery. Ellen knows me well enough to know how raw I was coming into the retreat. I am not one who cries much and yet I found myself on the verge of tears going into that retreat. I knew that Ellen would use her gift of nurturing to help get me through the retreat which would contain healing and other hard stuff.

This particular retreat consisted of a Friday night introductory session with a full day on Saturday and a closing session on Sunday morning. The Friday night session had gone pretty well and the audience was quite receptive and supportive as they found out the circumstances I was facing. While I spoke, I had even choked up which was something I rarely did. That was the first realization that this was going to be a different sort of retreat for me.

The next morning, Ellen and I were sitting at one of the big round tables which could seat about 6-

8 ladies. Over the years, I have found as a speaker that people are sometimes intimidated to talk or sit with me. In such situations, I strive to be engaging and inviting so that I can get to know others. However, given the events of the last few weeks, I was not at the top of my social game. But fortunately, for me, the four ladies who sat down at the table with Ellen and me did not know that.

Enter Judy and her daughters, Lori and Tara, and her daughter-in-law, Traci. Lori had organized a girls' weekend for the four of them and they were staying at her cabin near the retreat center. Lori was the only one of her group who attended Foothills and she was not part of the retreat planning committee. In addition, they had missed the Friday night session so none of them had any idea when they sat down with Ellen and me that I was the retreat speaker.

From the moment the six of us began talking, we found several connections. In addition to a shared love of the Lord, we shared many common interests as individuals. Ellen and Judy immediately began comparing grandchildren stories while Lori and I were both Boise State University alumni where I was teaching at the time. Ellen, Traci and I had all played softball although Traci left the two of us in the dust as she had played college softball. The common bond between Tara and I was my other alma mater, the University of Idaho, where she had attended about ten years after I had left.

Laughter and love became the common themes that ran through our interactions as a group. As a speaker, I had my own instant personal heckling section in Ellen, Judy, Lori, Tara and Traci. Laughter is good for the soul and mine had a wonderful workout over the course of the weekend! I laughed so hard that I was crying at times.

And other times throughout the weekend, I was crying without laughing not only because of Mom's death and Paul's illness but also the topic of friendship. As I have dealt with the dysfunction in my own family, my friends have become even more important to me. As I spoke, I was overwhelmed as I talked about how my friends had supported me through some of my most difficult times. Through misty eyes, I would look at the table of Ellen and my new friends and see supportive looks and praying going on while I shared my heart. That was only the beginning as the next few months and years unfolded.

"Let's do lunch" is an often overused and "under meant" term in our society. The phrase is social code for pretending that you want to get together with somebody when you really have no intention of doing so. Well in the case of the six of us, we meant it but knew that juggling schedules would be a challenge. Also, Traci would not be able to join us as she lived in southwest Oregon and coming ten hours for lunch in Boise was a bit of a stretch.

Nearly four months passed before the five of us found a date and time that would fit everybody's schedules. Tara suggested a centrally located Mexican restaurant near her office and we agreed to meet. Lori had picked up her kindergarten-aged daughter, Stacia, just before lunch and brought her along to join us. When they arrived at the restaurant,

Lori and Stacia sat down by me at one end of the long table.

Although five years old, Stacia kept up with and interjected into the conversation. She demonstrated that like her Mom, grandmother and aunts, she was intelligent and funny. We talked about her new glasses and her kindergarten basketball team and when I teased her, she returned the favor. As our lunch ended, we talked about getting back together and having Stacia and Tara's daughter join us as well.

God has a way of preparing us for the challenges we are to face and little did any of us know what was ahead just a few weeks later for Stacia. Doctors found that she had a cancerous brain tumor and removed it two days after Valentine's Day. In a flash, Stacia's world of basketball and kindergarten became one of doctors, hospitals and treatment options.

Lori and her husband Mike have an amazing and vast network of people supporting them through Stacia's diagnosis, surgery and treatment. I was one of about twenty people who were in the surgery waiting room with Mike, Lori and their son Bryce. We breathed a collective sigh of relief when Stacia not only survived the surgery, but doctors were able to remove the entire tumor. The real challenges had just begun as Stacia next faced 14 months of radiation and chemotherapy.

Through the course of my life, I have learned two valuable skills which have helped me minister to others who are in a health crisis. When I was in high school, my aunt and cousin were driving to a movie and were hit by a drunk driver. My aunt broke her leg and jaw while my cousin was in a coma for several days. During their hospitalization, my mom taught me how to stay with somebody who was recovering from illness or injury. She advised me that a sick person does not always want to talk so bring a book or something to do. Furthermore, Mom counseled to let them steer the conversation and level of activity. If a doctor, nurse or other caretaker entered the room, Mom said to find out if you needed to stay or leave and behave accordingly.

The other skill I learned was that a serious illness was often for the long-haul and most people, if they came at all, figured that the person was doing better much sooner than was actually true. This realization came to me as my friends began losing their parents or other loved ones. In our instant society, grieving was to occur quickly and be done faster than was reasonably expected. I would tell mourners that I would check back with them in a few months and beyond as that is usually when most all other folks would disappear.

So, I signed up for the long haul with Stacia and her family. I knew that many others would cover their meal needs at home and that was not my forte (although I am a pretty good baker). What I did know was that I did fine in hospitals so I began calling Lori to see if I could bring lunch or coffee to them while Stacia was having treatment. Sometimes I would drop off the food or beverage and go, but other times I would hang out and chat with the family or Lori and I would go find a corner and talk.

During those other times, Lori and I had some deep conversations. We had many things in common including a desire to be real and a love of the Lord. Those core principles became the foundation for our capacity to "speak the truth in love" into each other's lives. At that point, I was doing most of the speaking and Lori was doing much of the listening. The roles would be reversed when I had my cancer diagnosis and treatment.

The 14 months through which Stacia had her successful treatment were some of the most meaningful times of my life. I was honored to earn enough of Stacia's trust to be allowed to visit her at the hospital and at home. She kicked my butt at Wii more than any other person has ever done! Stacia slowly let me into her world and I learned a lot about how to deal with my cancer from this amazing kindergartener.

One side effect of her brain tumor was that Stacia could no longer write with her right hand. She did not whine and complain but rather started writing with her left hand. When she had to give up basketball, Stacia took up horseback riding. Again, no whining and complaining but rather adjusting to what was happening to her. When life gives us lemons, Stacia reminded me to make lemonade. After all, when life gave her cancer, Stacia made cancerade.

But when Stacia had her bad days as we all do, Lori received much of the brunt of this tough little girl who was also very scared and in pain. Her Dad, Mike, and brother, Bryce were very involved in Stacia's cancer treatment but were at work and school respectively for much of the time. In addition, Lori's parents were regularly involved.

As I said, I firmly believe that the Lord puts people in our lives at times when we need them. Such divine appointments may occur quickly such as the stranger who stops to help change a flat tire or says an encouraging word during a time of discouragement. Other times, those connections take root months or even years before. Being able to see those more long-term interactions gives us an opportunity to see God's Hand in an even more amazing way.

When I went to that women's retreat in the fall of 2009, I had no idea that I was having a divine appointment that would result in a crucial lifetime friendship. For just four months after Stacia successfully completed her cancer treatment, the shoe was on the other foot. I had cancer and I needed help. So, I turned to Lori to be the Captain of my Boundary Buddies. Blessedly, she took on the role without hesitation.

Within a day of my diagnosis, Lori and I were having coffee and she was giving me all sorts of welcome resources and advice. She thought about all sorts of issues and we began processing them to come up with workable solutions.

Lori's wisdom showed itself early on with a very important aspect of my cancer journey: communication. I did not want to spend valuable energy repeating the story of my cancer diagnosis, how I was doing and what the treatment was going to be. In addition, I grew up in a prominent Idaho family including politicians, physicians, attorneys, community activists and other prominent people. Being a member of the Hansen family opened many doors for me in life although once I entered, I had to prove myself on my own merits.

However, the experience also taught me a lot about communication. When something went right or wrong in my family, the incident would often appear in the newspaper or other media source. Living the public life made us the target of gossip and while I know that people will always gossip, I have learned that the best antidote is the truth in the hands of folks who would counteract the gossipers.

So I wanted to make sure the truth about my cancer was known to help squelch any rumors disguised as gossip and Lori had a terrific solution: CaringBridge.org. This terrific and free service allows people to keep loved ones informed in the case of a serious illness. CaringBridge helps minimize having to respond to each concerned person on an individual basis. Through Stacia's illness, Lori and Mike both posted on CaringBridge to keep their loved ones and others informed.

Lori and I talked through the logistics of using CaringBridge to let people know how I was faring and what I needed. We decided that I would set up the website and start posting about my cancer journey. As we got closer to the surgery and at the times I did not feel like posting, Lori would write about what was happening with my cancer journey.

In addition, Lori began going with me to my doctors' appointments and helped me get ready for them by preparing a list of questions I should ask. I would review the list and add to them as I thought of additional inquiries. Then, Lori would use my notebook to write down the answers to the questions as well as taking notes on what the doctors and nurses had said. The system worked very well as I could focus on the appointment and not have to be concerned about getting all of the information that was being provided to me.

The first major hurdle I had to clear was to figure out when to have the surgery. Lori had accompanied me to my appointment with Dr. Rudstad, the surgeon who had been recommended by Dr. Christensen. Like Drs. Nona and Christensen, Dr Rudstad is definitely a category 1 doctor (good doctoring skills and good communication skills). His knowledge of current practices was impressive from the first meeting and I knew I was in very good hands. He recommended a thyroidectomy (removal of my thyroid) and I took his advice.

I was diagnosed with papillary thyroid cancer which was relatively slow growing and only one tumor was determined at the time of my diagnosis to be cancerous. Neither the malignant tumor nor the one that was suspicious were near the 2.0 centimeter size that generated concern about possible spreading. The malignant tumor was 1.0 centimeter, the other tumor was about 6 millimeters and my peppered pals across the bottom half of my thyroid were not even big enough to measure. Furthermore, the cancer showed no signs of having spread to my lymph nodes. As I mentioned before, the bottom line was that my cancer had been caught very early and I had time on my side.

So, I decided to wait a couple of months to have my surgery and Dr. Rudstad said I could do so. I could take time to get my affairs in order and to make informed decisions without the pressure of having to have immediate surgery. I was so fortunate to have time on my side and am in continued awe of people like Lori and Mike who had to make quick decisions about Stacia's cancer treatment.

Lori and I synced up our schedules along with Dr. Rudstad and determined that November 30 would be the best date to have my surgery. I would be staying at Lori and Mike's home the night before I went into the hospital and for a week or so after I was released. In addition, I was in the midst of a book tour and wanted to make the most of that opportunity. Holiday sales are crucial in the book world and if I missed them, my bottom line would suffer significantly. Plus I had 50 authors who were part of the book and had been planning its release for months.

Also, I wanted to get myself as spiritually, physically, mentally and emotionally ready as possible for the surgery and treatment. I knew enough about cancer that the toll it can take on a person is greater than often suspected. I needed to deal with the emotions that I was feeling and prepare myself to take some time off after the surgery. Issues like my will and powers of attorney which had been languishing on my to-do list suddenly shot to the top of my priority list. In addition, I have a family history of heart problems and wanted to make sure that I received the all-clear from a cardiologist.

My decision to wait was not well received by some people in my life. I was advised to deal with the feelings later and get the surgery done now. Although I disagreed with her, I appreciated the honesty of my friend who said that to me because most folks were not that direct. In addition, I remember running into one person in a grocery store parking lot who wanted to know why I was waiting two months to have my surgery.

"Do you have to wait for the tumor to get bigger before you have it removed?" she asked.

"No," I replied and got to the heart of her question. "I am waiting because I can."

Actually, I appreciated this woman's candor even if she did not directly ask me why I was waiting. Over the years, I have learned to appreciate and to develop candor in my life. Learning to be open and honest was a skill I honed and one that continues to help me through my life particularly as I faced my thyroid cancer. However, developing that skill took study and practice as secret keeping was a fixture of my growing up.

EGGSHELLS AND ELEPHANTS

From the moment I decided to write a book about my cancer, journey, I knew that the title would be "Eggshells and Elephants" as my illness involved a lot of walking on eggshells and recognizing the elephants in the living room. The first phrase "walking on eggshells" refers to gently stepping through a particular situation: in other words, eggshells are very fragile and could easily break if stepped on too hard. You would "walk on eggshells" around a sensitive person or subject to avoid causing hurt feelings, arguments and the like. A related phrase would be "walking through a minefield" which can be even more dangerous as eggshells can most often be seen while mines usually cannot. In addition, mines explode.

The other metaphor is "the elephant in the living room" and that has to do with an obvious issue that people do not want to discuss. If you have an elephant in your living room, you and anybody else in your home would be hard-pressed to ignore it. However if the subject is touchy or controversial, most folks will opt to not talk about it; that is, ignore the elephant in the living room.

These metaphors are particularly meaningful to me because I spent my growing up living with them as part of my reality. You see, my parents were AMAZING human beings. As previously mentioned, Dad was born in Austria and escaped the Holocaust. On the other hand, my mom survived the Depression living with her parents and five brothers in the basement of a house on the outskirts of Idaho Falls.

Despite all they had been through with their growing up, Mom and Dad accomplished a great deal. They both earned college degrees as did all six of their children. Mom and Dad both coached sports teams of young people and encouraged community involvement. I will always be thankful as Mom and Dad gave me my education, taught me a lifelong love of learning, and showed me how to give back to my community.

However, my parents were very human. My mom was a gifted teacher, the best conversationalist I have ever met, a puppeteer who gave puppets to kids in abusive situations and was an active alcoholic until the day she died. Mom's drinking occurred in the evening after work so her alcoholism was not apparent to many people outside of our family or so I thought. As I became older and discussed the subject with childhood friends, I was surprised to find out that they all knew Mom was an alcoholic because their parents knew. The elephant in the living room was standing in front of a big picture window.

On the other hand, my dad was a brilliant chemical and nuclear engineer who got his bachelors and masters degrees from MIT (Massachusetts Institute of Technology) in five years, could explain nuclear energy to children, was a talented coach, and was chronically depressed and had two nervous breakdowns in the course of his life.

The irony is that Dad's depression was likely connected to his thyroid cancer. The level of the thyroid function is related to depression and Dad's thyroid was not functioning correctly for longer than anybody on this Earth knew. Furthermore, chronic depression can lead to nervous breakdowns particularly if the true source of the problem is not being treated as was the case with Dad's depression.

For many years, Dad would go in for his annual physical which included the doctor palpitating Dad's thyroid. Well, all those years his doctors were "feeling Dad's thyroid', they were in fact way off of the mark. Turns out that Dad's thyroid was actually at the base of his throat; a fact that was not discovered until his thyroid cancer was so advanced that it had paralyzed one of Dad's vocal cords.

In April 1998, my siblings and I arrived in Idaho Falls for Grandma Hansen's funeral to discover that Dad would be having thyroid cancer surgery the day after her services. Amazingly, doctors got 90% of Dad's cancer which had spread to his lymph nodes, chest wall, esophagus, epiglottis and trachea. Radiation got the last 10% and the only long-term physical problem Dad had was that his epiglottis never functioned correctly after that and he spent the last few years of his life on a feeding tube. Despite the advanced state of Dad's cancer, that was not what killed him. He died in 2006 at the age of 78 of congestive heart failure.

Research shows that 90-95% of American families have some level of dysfunction and that the rest still have issues, but they have learned to communicate through them. I believe my family fell right into the midst of the dysfunctional statistic and were living amongst eggshells and elephants.

Now I came to these realizations in the form of hindsight which is 20/20. Only much later in life did I learn about dysfunction and how to deal with it.

A life-changing book for me was "Adult Children: Secrets of Dysfunctional Families" by John and Linda Friel. This book helped me name what I had been through and if you can name it, you can claim it and that is exactly what I did.

While I was at home, I made attempts to deal with the eggshells and elephants head on. When I was 18, while I was home from college on spring break, I sat down with my mom on the porch and told her I thought she had a drinking problem. The main lesson I learned was to never say, "I think you have a drinking problem" to somebody who has been drinking as Mom had been at that point. She was understandably upset and did not take my comments well. Our relationship suffered for quite some time as we were both very hurt.

On the other hand, a very positive thing happened in our relationship as suddenly we were able to talk about a lot of subjects we had never previously discussed. After all, the "alcoholism elephant" was now in plain sight so we could discuss that and other issues in our lives. Mom and I shared parts of our lives that we shared with nobody else.

Dad's depression and nervous breakdowns also had a positive impact on our relationship. Besides the obvious father-daughter relationship, Dad and I shared another bond: brown eyes. In fact, I am the only one of Mom and Dad's children to share brown eyes like Dad. His nickname for me was "Brown Eyes", a term of endearment that I greatly appreciate.

Not only did we share brown eyes but also similar personalities, enjoyment of analyzing and senses of humor. Add that to my education in psychology and communication and Dad and I would have some great discussions and could get to the heart of the matter with his depression. I believe that the most useless knowledge is that which stays in the classroom. In other words, discussion without practical application is pretty pointless. So when Dad and I talked about his depression, we would not only analyze what was happening but come up with concrete things we could do to help him out.

One piece of advice that I gave him and have shared with many others struggling with depression is "What is one thing you can do today that you did not do yesterday?" Some days that means going outside and some days that means getting out of bed. Having a reasonable goal like that gives somebody with depression an opportunity to see out of the black hole they can find themselves in.

Through their alcoholism and depression, Mom and Dad showed me how to work through the tough stuff. Please understand that having alcoholism and depression play such big roles in my growing up was no walk in the park. I have gone through counseling and other recovery work to help me put what I have been through in perspective. However, I have seen many benefits to what the Lord walked me through via the challenges of my childhood. My experience has allowed me to help others through similar challenges. The fact that I studied psychology and communication and taught the latter is directly related to wanting to understand what I had gone through and to change how I had been affected.

Another very important lesson I learned is best summed up by Oswald Chambers in his classic book "My Utmost for His Highest" when he said in his June 17 devotional: "There is always at least one more fact, which we know nothing about, in every person's situation." In other words, I never know what elephant is in somebody else's living room but need to be aware there's one if not more there.

Like any other challenge in my life, I had two choices: wallow in it or work through it. I tried the wallowing for a while and found little benefit in doing so. So, I decided to work through it and am a better person for having done so.

When people ask me how I managed to come through what I have and be relatively unscathed, I credit three things for having done so: 1) Jesus Christ is my Lord and Savior and the center of my life. 2) I was willing to talk about what I had been through and 3) I developed significant relationships outside my family from an early age.

Speaking of which, those significant relationships in the forms of friendships and family members were or were not a major part of my thyroid cancer journey. As has been the case with many momentous events in my life, I am surprised who has supported me and I am surprised who has not. Whether the occasion was being elected student body president in college, accepting Jesus Christ as my Lord and Savior, or becoming an author and a publisher, I have had people come out of the woodwork to support me and had some who were close to me turn away.

I found that people fell into different categories in terms of relating to me about my cancer diagnosis. The first group consisted of people who were either walking on eggshells around me or acted like my cancer was the elephant in the living room. The second group was people who talked openly about my cancer and acknowledged what I was going through. They could say or hear the word "cancer" and not cringe, choke or gasp.

However with my cancer I had an added twist as there was a third category of people: those who I temporarily backed away from. I had to focus my physical, emotional, spiritual and mental energy on getting better and not on hand-holding people who could not handle the fact that I had cancer. The time to return to those relationships came when I was feeling better. I felt no guilt about my decisions as I knew that my cancer had to be about me. As I told a longtime friend as we were discussing some of the "backlash" I was getting: "I know how to ask for help and I will do it in the ways I need help. If folks are ready to help, that's great but if they're not then get out of my way."

Although those in the first two groups differed on their ability to talk about "cancer", many people in these groups bent over backwards to do what they could to help. Some people could not say "I love you" but could show it. The bottom line was these folks were showing that they cared in the ways they were able to do so; they simply chose different ways to communicate their concerns. However, such assistance came in a variety of forms and sometimes involves walking on eggshells.

Mark 2:1-12 tells the story of the dedication of four friends to their pal who was paralyzed. Jesus was at the height of his popularity and was at a home in Capernaum. So many people came to see Him that no room was available in the house. However, these four friends knew that if they got their paralytic pal to Jesus that he would be healed. They put their friend on the mat, climbed up on top of the house, cut a hole in the roof, and lowered the mat down. Jesus healed the man who then rolled up his mat and walked out of the home.

Sometimes in life, we are on the mat and sometimes, we are carrying the mat. Having good balance in life is knowing when to get on the mat and when to let others carry you. With my cancer journey, I was on the mat. In some areas of my cancer journey, I accepted help in many forms However in other facets, I had some very definite ideas about the help I needed and the help I did no.

Personally, I am prone to making food for people who are sick, having a bad day or are some combination of down. So, I recognize that some people do the same thing. Along my cancer journey, I needed food but not in the ways that many folks wanted to provide it. For example, well-meaning cooks would make meals that fed more than one person. That's a very polite way of saying most meals for the sick could feed a small army. Since I am the only human in my home and have a small freezer, home-cooked meals were not the answer.

This dilemma was one of the many times that Lori's experience with Stacia's cancer was helpful to me: Lori came up with idea for gift cards to some of my favorite restaurants. I could have food delivered or picked up and order meals for just me, myself and

I. Brilliant solution but not one that everybody embraced so that's when Captain Lori intervened on my behalf.

Lori posted the following very well-worded message on my CaringBridge site: "Please remember that one of the best ways Jane has indicated you can help is by providing her meal gift cards to some of her favorite places. She does not have the space for prepared meals, and she also knows how much "leftover" food can come with prepared meals." The message accomplished its goal as I received a whole bunch of gift cards.

However I had dear friends actually tell me that "No, you are going to want a home cooked meal." Pretty gutsy from my perspective as I was the one with the cancer. I politely explained that we could enjoy a home cooked meal together down the road after I had recovered, but during the immediate time post surgery, gift cards would be best.

I will admit that such conversations frustrated me as demonstrated by the condition of my favorite tennis shoes. When the conversation was nerve-wracking but was not worth the battle, I would curl my toes in my shoes. As a result, I ended up blowing out the sides of my sneakers by the time I was home from the hospital.

I did particularly appreciate the friends with whom I could be totally honest. I remember one friend who called me to find out when she could bring meals by and I did not get her called back immediately. Being one of the most organized people I know, she had the meals prepared by the time I contacted her back. When she asked about bringing them by, I took a deep breath and explained my freezer dilemma.

"Not a problem, Jane," she replied. "My husband and I can freeze the meals and eat them over time. We have plenty of freezer space."

"Thank you so much," I said with an obvious tone of relief in my voice.

She chuckled. "Having your fill of helpful people?"

I laughed and said, "You hit that nail on the head!" I am so very thankful as I have been blessed with some amazing friendships with people who care more than I could ever imagine. I received some very lovely notes, e-mails, cards, gifts, letters and other contacts which touched me in very special ways. One benefit of my cancer was that I got a very good taste of what people thought of me (kind of like going to my own funeral without having to die).

Speaking of funerals, the final piece of advice I will share in this chapter about being a friend to somebody in crisis came from attending a memorial service. My college friend's brother had been killed in a hunting accident while we were still in school. At that point in my life, I was a novice about attending funerals as I had gone to only a handful of such services.

At the cemetery after the burial, I hung back from offering condolences to the family as I did not know what to say. Finally, I got up the nerve and went to my friend. I hugged her, offered my sympathies and said that I almost did not come up to the family as I was not sure what to say.

"Come up anyway," she said. "Being there is what is most important."

Whether you write an encouraging note, call to chat, pray (including for the caregivers), send flowers or other gifts, visit the person in crisis, or do some other kind act, do something (AKA being there) as that means so much to somebody who is facing a health crisis. I know from first-hand experience of being on both sides of that coin just how much that thoughtfulness means.

But I also I learned first-hand that when a person has a major illness or other crisis, it's about that individual and not about me. If I have expectations of a certain response from the person who is sick, then I am making the illness about me. My only expectation of somebody facing a health crisis is they focus on themselves and getting better. If I find myself offended by their response or lack thereof, I need to check my motives.

Now having said all that and in my cancer journey, I know that people almost always mean well and that's what really counts. A health crisis in somebody they care about can rock their world and showing some grace is much easier on all involved.

DETAILS, DETAILS, DETAILS

By nature, I am not an organized person and details have not been my strong suit. That fact became very apparent to me several years ago when I decided that I had too many books and should donate and sell those I was not reading nor had any intention to do so. In the process, I found three different books on organizing. Not a good sign so I decided to make getting and staying organized a priority of mine.

I began by hiring a young person to organize my remaining books into topics and then by author. She did an outstanding job of getting them in order so much so that I ended up finding more books to give away. Next, I went through my files and kept what I needed and discarded what I did not. I developed the attitude of "What would I want people to have to deal with when I die?" So, when in doubt I threw it out (actually I gave it away but that does not rhyme with "when in doubt"!)

Over the years, I have made a lot of change in my life: overcoming shyness, starting a business, walking with the Lord and the list goes on and on. Throughout these transitions, I have used two strategies: observation and education. In terms of getting organized, I have picked up tips by observing people who are more organized than I am and by educating myself through books and articles on the subject. Life is easier when I do not have to reinvent the wheel.

But at the core of making change is attitude and having a good one about being organized helped me as I was facing all of the details related to my thyroid cancer. As with any surgery or major illness, the possibility of dying or becoming disabled is very real and I had the family history to show it.

The only one of my grandparents I ever knew was my maternal grandma. As I mentioned earlier, my Dad's parents died when he was six weeks old (Grandma Freund) and about seven (Grandpa Freund). Dad had little memory of his dad and no memory of his mom. On the other hand, Mom knew both her parents as Grandma Hansen lived to be almost 97, but her dad died much sooner than that. When Mom was a freshman in college, Grandma and Grandpa Hansen were sitting by the fireplace enjoying a quiet Sunday night in November 1949. Grandpa reached over to put a log on the fire and collapsed from a cerebral hemorrhage. He never regained consciousness and died within a day. Grandpa was just 47 and his only grandchild he ever knew was but a few weeks old.

Grandma Hansen found herself with a family farm, an auto dealership, and three children in college, Along with her six children, Grandma had to work hard to make it but they did. Interestingly, Grandma had to give up the auto dealership because "in those days", the Ford Motor Company would not let a woman own such a business.

Fast forward ahead just over 55 years to another experience that taught me a great deal about getting one's affairs in order. As I said before, a few months after Dad died, my brother Paul (P.D.) was diagnosed with a good-sized benign brain tumor and surgery was performed. During the procedure, Paul had a stroke and spent over two weeks (including his

40th birthday) in a coma. P.D. awoke from his coma but never returned to his home and is now in a long-term care facility.

I learned from Grandpa Hansen's death and Paul's disability respectively to make sure that all of my affairs were in order. Details such as powers of attorney, will, funeral arrangements, care of animals, distribution of property and other things had to be spelled out. I refused to be naïve and think that death and disability were out of the realm of my possibility. Better to have peace of mind than to make others guess what I wanted.

Also, Grandpa and Paul's experiences resulted in me taking an extra step. Besides thyroid cancer, my family medical history includes heart problems with both Mom and Dad having congestive heart failure and Dad dying of the disease. Although I had no symptoms of heart problems, I asked my doctor to refer me to a cardiologist to make absolutely certain I did not have a hidden issue which would show its ugly head during my surgery. He did not hesitate and sent me to a heart doctor.

In addition to my family heart health history, I had two other reasons for wanting my ticker checked out. First of all, heart disease is the number one cause of death of women in the United States. Second, I had no warning that I had thyroid cancer and did not want a repeat performance with heart disease. Thankfully, the cardiologist gave me the all clear to go ahead and have the surgery. I certainly appreciate what my parents, Grandpa Hansen and P.D. taught me through their illnesses.

Speaking of which, I proceeded with getting all of my affairs in order. Fortunately, I have a very stellar attorney who walked me through the process of getting my medical and financial powers of attorney in place as well as making sure my will was written to my specifications. I did have to think about things I had not considered such as who would get my dogs and cats, my business and very specific pieces of my personal property.

However, I knew that I had to be very deliberate about my choice of people to make sure that my wishes were carried through. Fortunately, the two people I asked to take on the roles were willing to do so and individuals with whom I could have the tough conversations. One was Captain Lori of the Boundaries Bunch and the other was my friend Rebecca. I have told you how I connected with Lori so let me share how Rebecca became a very dear Freund, I mean friend of mine.

The slip in the last paragraph was deliberate because Rebecca's maiden name is Freund. Nothing too unusual about that except that for many years I knew only one other Freund family in all of Idaho. But now that Idaho has grown significantly in population with over one million people in the Gem State, more Freunds can be found here.

In the case of Rebecca, we met when we were both working for a company that helped people with developmental disabilities. Rebecca worked full-time while the sum total of my hours were in the neighborhood of 3-4 weekly as I helped run a Friday night social group for teenage clients. This fact is significant because of the small size of my paycheck (about $25-30 every two weeks) and how it led to my connecting with Rebecca.

The company offered the service of directly depositing our paychecks so I signed up. After a couple of my "huge" checks did not end up in my account, I did some checking and found out that my paychecks had been inadvertently deposited in Rebecca's account. I saw this as a good opportunity to meet this other Freund and find out how she had come to Idaho. I took said opportunity at a company staff meeting.

Having had somebody point Rebecca out to me, I went up to her at said, "Hey, you stole my paycheck." Now remember that Rebecca did not know me from Eve and add to that the fact that our personalities are a bit different: I am more extroverted and she is more introverted.

The look on Rebecca's face was priceless as she was clearly surprised and did not know what to say. While she stumbled for some words, I explained who I was and what had happened. We both had a good laugh and the incident became the start of a terrific friendship. Oh and Rebecca and her family came to Idaho when her dad became pastor of a church in the southern Idaho town of Buhl. That piece of information is interesting because that's the same town where Lori grew up and yet she and Rebecca did not know each other until I introduced them.

I chose Lori and Rebecca because I know they both love the Lord and I could have the very difficult conversations with them. In this case, the discussion was the "what to do if I die or become disabled" one.

I had and still have no doubt that they would carry out my wishes and I made those instructions perfectly clear. While such topics can be hard to contemplate and to discuss, doing so is the correct road to take and amazing peace of mind is the result.

On the other hand, I planned for the distinct possibility that I would recover from surgery and come home. (NOTE: that is what happened as indicated by the fact that this book is not written posthumously by somebody else). Those plans were much easier to make as they involved leaving for an extended period of time and coming home, something I had done many times before.

Many years ago, I discovered that the last thing I wanted to do when I came back after a trip was to deal with a dirty home. So, I made a point of changing my beds, emptying the dishwasher, cleaning out the fridge, vacuuming, dusting and otherwise prepping for my return before I left. Doing so meant that I could climb into bed or plop down on the couch and relax when I got home. That strategy is a keeper.

The next issue was to make sure that the dogs and cats had appropriate care. My cats, Curtis, Theolonius and Hummer were veterans of this process as I had found a dear friend, Mary Anne, who would come over and take care of them on a daily basis. A cat lover herself, Mary Anne bonded with my felines including the somewhat skittish Hummer who now refers to Mary Anne as her BFF.

On the other hand, Moose and Mickey would have to go to the kennel because they do not do well without regular human attention and they refuse to use the litter box. Thankfully, I had found a wonderful place to board them and Moose and Mickey enjoy going there.

So, I made the appropriate animals arrangements including a list of veterinarians, kennels, medical conditions and feeding instructions. In addition, I provided extra cat litter, food and funds; the latter of which in case the former two ran out. Mary Anne even graciously agreed to water my house plants since the cats refused to do so.

In terms of financial considerations, I made sure my bills were paid ahead of time. Also, I arranged for my mail to be picked up from my post office boxes, any checks deposited and book orders fulfilled which was particularly important at the holiday season.

Details, details, details...all taken care of (or so I thought).

FLEEING FLEAS

One of my favorite sayings is "People plan and God laughs". Well, He was getting a pretty good chuckle out of me when I thought I had taken care of all of the details needed before I would have my thyroid cancer surgery. Despite all of my best efforts, little did I know that my darling dogs would require some extra attention prior to my surgery.

For as long as I can remember, I grew up with dogs. While I have vague memories of our other dogs prior to her, Patches was our first canine with whom I really bonded. My parents had decided to get a boxer and were particularly interested in the two white boxer puppies the breeder had in the litter. Because of the desire to make the boxer breed more pure, this breeder "should" have destroyed these two white boxer puppies. But, fortunately he was a true dog lover and did not murder the puppies.

Mom and Dad decided to buy one of the two white boxer puppies. Because they had six children in the house, my parents requested the gentler of the two puppies. Well according to our family lore, the breeder decided that with such a big family that we would need protection. He sold Mom and Dad the more aggressive of the two puppies (a fact that my parents did not know at the time). So when I was just six years old, Patches came to be part of our family.

Patches was totally white with the exception of two brown patches: one over her eye and one by her stubby tail. Some of my siblings and I suggested that we name the dog "Lily" because she was white and Grandma Hansen was named Lily. In one of her many wise insights, Mom steered us toward the name "Patches" as she correctly recognized that Grandma would NOT be thrilled to have a dog named after her.

And what a dog Patches grew into being! She had a classic boxer look with a barrel chest and wiry legs and oh was she strong! Patches would crack cow knucklebones in her jaw. My brother would have tug of wars with her using a string of athletic socks tied together and Patches more than held her own.

Patches also had an iron constitution. In sixth grade, we were reading "Jonah and the Whale" and had to carve a whale out of Ivory soap as an assignment. Well in a true classic case of "my dog ate my homework", Patches got to my whale carving and chewed it up pretty badly. When I told my teacher the next day, I could tell that he did not quite believe me. So I went home and dug what remained of my whale out of the garbage and took it to school the next day. I set the half-chewed whale carving completed with dried dog slobber and hair on my teacher's desk. His response was priceless: "Good gravy! Your dog really did eat your homework!" I ended up getting full credit for the assignment.

Speaking of food, Patches had a personality all her own. When we would have family dinner, she would go in the backroom and eat her food. Well, Patches was putting on some weight so my folks bought her some diet dog food. While dog food has progressed significantly since then, diet dog food in the 1970s was often pretty nasty and Patches proved that point.

When Patches ate, her collar and tags would clang against her metal bowl so between that and her snorting, it was pretty obvious when Patches was eating. Well the first time Patches had that diet dog food, the noise was a bit different. First, Patches ate some of the food and then the metal bowl could be heard sliding across the linoleum floor. A small "crash" was heard followed by more metal crossing with linoleum and then a big "CRASH" with a bunch of smaller sounds of what sounded like pebbles being scattered. Upon investigation, we found that Patches had pushed her bowl of diet dog food down the basement stairs. She let it be known how little she thought of that food so we gave the remaining bag to our friends to feed their black lab, Liz, who scarfed it down. Not too surprising as Liz was the same dog who would entertain us by catching sand in her mouth thus demonstrating she would eat pretty much anything.

However, the other side of Patches' personality did show and that was her dislike of men outside of our immediate family. The only non-Freund man I remember Patches liking was my Uncle Reed, one of my Mom's brothers. Patches demonstrated her dislike for non-family males with actions such as grabbing a wrist without biting as if to say, "I do not like you doing that so do not do it again". I learned a lot about nonverbal communication from Patches.

I experienced the gentler side of Patches and she was a major reason I have a lifelong connection to animals. Patches was my companion when I would go sit under a tree and read for hours. The two of us would go for walks or play in our big yard. My parents were concerned that Patches would stunt my growth because she slept across my legs at night. Simply put, Patches was a terrific first dog to have in my life.

With life, unfortunately, comes death and so came the end of Patches' time on Earth. When I was about 15, Patches started having seizures. At first I was scared when they happened but then would sit with her and repeat "Patches Poochy Baby" which was my nickname for her.

The vet examined Patches and determined she either had epilepsy or a brain tumor (the latter could explain her aggressive personality). He said that the tests he needed to run to figure out which illness was plaguing Patches would kill her. So, we made the agonizing decision to put her to sleep. Dad and I took Patches to the vet and I still remember saying goodbye to her. We had an amazing bond.

Over the years that followed, we had other cool dogs, but when I became an adult, I found cats to be easier to have because they did not require as much attention. With the exception of a stray dog I had found a home for many years ago, I had not had dogs in my life for about 25 years until Moose and Mickey came to live with me.

One trait Mom and I shared was a love of animals and a deep bond with them. With that in mind, years ago, I had promised Mom that I would take her Shih-tzus, Moose and Mickey, if they outlived her. These dogs were particularly special as they had kept Mom company after Dad went into the nursing home and died a year or so later. When Mom herself became homebound due to poor health, Moose and

Mickey kept her going when she was discouraged. Moose and Mickey did not care if Mom did not feel like letting them out and would scratch at the door until she responded accordingly.

However in the case of Moose and Mickey, "dogs" is a relative term. Mom referred to them as "the boys" and with good reason: I do not think that Moose and Mickey knew they were dogs. The biggest clue to that was that every night they lived with Mom and Dad and then Mom alone, Moose and Mickey, each got their own fresh cooked marrow bone. Mom's caregivers knew which grocery stores had the bones for sale on what days as they were a very precious commodity. Often when I visited Idaho Falls, I too would make trips to buy the bones and cook them up.

Well in September 2009 after Mom died, the daily marrow bones became a thing of the past when Moose and Mickey came to live with me in Boise. Mickey had a very rough time with the move as he was very close to Mom. For the first four months, his health was touch and go as he dealt with separation anxiety. Mom was with Moose and Mickey pretty much 24/7 through the last four years of her life. While I work out of my home, I would leave and that was especially difficult for Mickey. But, I learned a lot about dealing with his anxiety and he came to figure out that I would come back and was not leaving forever like Mom had done.

In addition, I had to introduce my cats, Curtis, Theolonius and Hummer to these "intruders" who were now part of our lives; quite the transition when Alpha Dog Mickey met Alpha Cat Curtis, who had treed raccoons and chased a black lab off my porch. Curtis would not be bothered with these yappy little creatures who were about his size and only spoke the foreign language of "WOOF". Over time, the dogs and cats negotiated a peace deal, but only after a few incidents such as Hummer biting off Mickey's toenail and one or both dogs chasing Theolonius up the tallest bookcase in my home. Now they all know I am in charge so things are much more peaceful

With five animals and all of them except Hummer being at least ten years old, I was on a first name basis with the staff at my vets' office. In the weeks prior to my cancer surgery, Moose was the one who required a few trips to the vets' office. He had been to the doggie doctor many times over his life particularly when he was about seven and ended up losing his eye to an infection. He has adapted well and has even been nicknamed "The Pirate Dog" by some of my friends.

But at this time, the problem was not Moose's eye but his skin. In late October about a month prior to my cancer surgery, he had developed pink welts on his underside and was scratching and licking his backside quite a bit. I took Mickey and Moose to the vet to make sure the latter was OK and because they are the epitome of canine codependence. Mickey was healthy, but the vet prescribed a steroid and an antibiotic for Moose. Over the course of the next few weeks, Moose's welts went away and his scratching and licking subsided.

After the medicine ran out, Moose's symptoms returned and so the Monday before Thanksgiving, I called the vets' office to make an appointment to have Moose looked at again. The doctor, who was best suited to see him, would not be in until Wednesday, the day before Thanksgiving. Again, I brought Mickey along so he would not need therapy after being away from Moose for an hour and of course to get him checked as well.

Despite my years of canine companionship, I had managed to dodge a major doggy problem until that fateful day I took Moose and Mickey to the vet. As I lifted Mickey up onto the examination table, I surprised myself by asking a question I had never faced before with any dog I had been around: "Could this be fleas?" The vet parted the hair on Mickey's back and the fleas were running across his skin. An examination of Moose's skin showed fleas as well. His welts were because he was allergic to the fleas.

The previous vet had goofed and missed the fleas. I was not interested in placing blame as I make mistakes too. In addition, I knew that I needed to take care of the flea problem immediately as my surgery was in just a week and a major holiday known as Thanksgiving cut back my "make the fleas flee" time even more.

I called the dog kennel and confirmed what I suspected: Moose and Mickey could not stay there if they had any signs of fleas. They were to be there the Tuesday after Thanksgiving and the day before my surgery. Also, my dog groomer would not let them in if they had fleas either and I certainly understood as providing fleas to other dogs is not good customer service. So, I had to come up with an alternative for getting Moose and Mickey's fleas gone ASAP.

The vets' staff jumped in and immediately offered to bathe Moose and Mickey to get rid of any fleas and eggs they could. They also provided me with medicine to give to the cats to deal with any fleas or eggs that were on their skin. While others may have success with bathing cats, I did not fall into that category and even have the scar to prove it.

Also, the staff instructed me how to flea bomb the house to rid the joint of fleas and eggs. I had heard stories of others who bombed their house and all of the extra effort that was involved in doing so. Plus, I did not like the idea of the cats having to breathe in those chemicals for seven days while they would be inside and I would be at the hospital and then staying at Lori and Mike's home.

So I did what I usually did when I needed answers and that was tap into my network of friends, acquaintances and family and what better way to do it than through Facebook. I posted that I was looking for some natural ways to deal with fleas and asked for suggestions. My friend, Noreen, recommended spreading salt and baking soda on the furniture and carpets, waiting 20 minutes or more and vacuuming all the surfaces. On my way home, I stopped at the grocery store and bought more baking soda and salt in one trip than I had purchased in the last several years.

The first step when I got home was to determine if the cats had fleas too. I examined their skin and found a little bit of flea dirt on Hummer, but Curtis and Theolonius were clean. If I was a flea, I would not mess with Curtis either; he chased raccoons up a tree so for heaven's sake he would not be afraid of a flea.

While the freshly sprinkled salt and baking soda did their work, I did mine and applied the flea medicine to the back of the cats' necks. Then, I vacuumed the furniture and carpets and began cleaning counters and every non-vacuum able surface in the house. By the time I was done, Thanksgiving was almost upon me and I prayed the fleas had fled. Oh if it was that simple.

The day after Thanksgiving, I called my vets' office and asked if they could pretty well shave Moose and Mickey. I figured that having most all of their hair gone would give the fleas less places to hide. I did not care how Moose and Mickey looked as that was not nearly as important as ridding them of the fleas. The vets' staff agreed to help out and did the best they could to cut Moose and Mickey's hair as short as possible.

In the end, Moose and Mickey would not have won any grooming awards as they looked like they had been attacked by a set of out-of-control clippers. However the plan worked and by the following Monday, Moose and Mickey were pronounced flea-free and could go to the kennel the next day for their week-long stay. I did not take much time to celebrate as within 48 hours, I would be having my cancer surgery.

The next day, Tuesday, was a blur as I had a lot of last minute things to get done including dropping the now flealess boys off at the kennel. Before I knew it, the day had disappeared and Lori was at my door to pick me up and take me to their home. I would spend the night and then before dawn even thought about cracking the next morning, I would be at the hospital. The time had come.

LIKELY

I slept relatively well the night before I went in for surgery because I had a pretty straightforward attitude: either I would survive the surgery or I would not and end up with the Lord. As far as I was concerned, the situation was win-win.

I was fortunate that I had done my hospital check-in about a week prior to the surgery. The thought of being coherent enough to answer detailed questions the morning of my surgery was not pleasant. Unfortunately, I had lost my check-in paperwork, but the admission folks were quite gracious and accommodated the burp in the process.

Soon I was in pre-op waiting while they put in the IV, took my blood pressure (and gave it back) as well as asking me a whole bunch of questions to ensure they were doing the correct procedure on the right person. With the horror stories I had heard about hospital mistakes, I was more than happy to repeat my name and birth date to each medical professional who walked into the prep area.

Soon, Lori came back to sit with me for moral support and to take notes on any important information. The drugs were beginning to take effect and I wanted to make sure I did not miss any crucial details. The wait took longer than expected as a problem had occurred with the airflow in the operating room. Surgeries that were already in progress were to be finished, but folks like me who were in the on-deck circle had to wait until the technicians could fix the problem.

As a result, we had more time to chat with the various medical personnel who stopped in to see how I was doing. When Dr. Rudstad came into the room, we talked and joked a bit more than usual. From the first appointment I had with him, I appreciated his straightforward approach and great bedside manner. As he wrapped up the conversation, he reviewed the procedure and my current condition. He referred to the two tumors as "cancerous" and "likely" and then went into more detail about what they would be doing. Then, he wished me well and walked out the door to prep for the surgery.

If you have ever seen the old Charlie Brown cartoons on television, you know that every adult sounds like "wah wah wah" to Charlie Brown and his friends. As I replayed in my mind I had just heard, suddenly everything sounded like "wah wah wah" except his reference to the tumors. The second tumor had gone from "probable" cancer to "likely" cancer. Most likely a question of semantics, but to me, I had crossed over to it "likely" being cancer which was like being on the other side of the cancer mountain. Instead of one cancer tumor, I likely had a second, albeit small, cancerous tumor.

I turned to Lori and asked if she had heard the change in terms on the second tumor. "Yes," she replied. I was more surprised and not mad at all by what he said as I still had cancer whether there were one or two tumors. Communication is not perfect and the fact that I did not know the true condition of the second tumor demonstrated that reality. The ballgame had changed, but I still needed to take my turn at bat whether I had one or two strikes against me. Just needed to know what I was facing.

Soon the technicians came to roll me out of pre-op and into surgery. I had not undergone general anesthesia since 1980 and that had had a very surprising result after an interesting beginning. About four weeks after I graduated high school and six weeks before I was to start college, I went in for my first gynecological examination. Oh joy, a pap smear I thought to myself, but I needed to have one on my next step to womanhood.

The doctor performed his examination and called in his nurse to be in the room while he talked with me. "You have an ovarian cyst," he explained.

Several years earlier, I had had a small cyst removed from the back of my head. I curled my forefinger into the base of my thumb and formed a dime-sized circle. "Cyst?" I questioned as I held up my thumb and finger in an appropriately sized circle to make my point.

"No. It's about the size of a soccer ball." he said calmly.

My head immediately went where no young person should ever have to go. "Is it cancer?" I asked.

"It's a one-in-three chance," he said as I watched my future quickly disappear.

The next morning I was in the hospital having tests run to determine the extent of the damage the cyst had caused my body. Initial reports indicated that my right kidney was not functioning properly; surgery the next day showed the lack of function was due to the fact that my right kidney did not exist.

Fortunately, my left kidney is larger than normal and functions well.

Surgery also showed that the cyst was not only benign but also not a cyst. Rather, the "growth" was a second uterus filled with blood because the organ was not fully opened. The surgeons, one of whom was my uncle, opened up the uterus and drained out the blood. Mine was the first case of uterine didelphius that either of the doctors had seen.

When I woke up that day, I asked my mom if I had cancer. She told me no and I went back to sleep. After the anesthesia wore off and I was more coherent, I told her that the drugs must have done a trick on my mind because I remembered being in surgery, then back in the operating room and then back into surgery.

"That's what happened because they left a tool inside you." She replied. The blood from my second uterus (AKA U2) had backed up into my stomach and doctors had used an abdominal blood cyst tool and then left it inside of me. They went back in and got it out.

So my last surgery over 32 years before had resulted in a medical mistake and phenomenon. I was hoping that my cancer surgery did not result in a repeat performance, but I had a new tool in my repertoire that I did not have at the time of the last surgery: I knew the peace of the Lord and that made a world of difference.

So rather than beginning my thyroidectomy surgery at 7:30 AM, I went in about 8:30 AM. I remember counting down in the operating room and then nothing until groggy memories of the recovery room. The surgery was scheduled to take between 1 1/2 to 2 hours assuming that no lymph node involvement existed. By 10:30 AM, the surgery was complete.

Fortunately, the surgery went very well. As expected, both of the tumors on the top of my thyroid were cancerous. The results on the peppered smaller tumors across the bottom of my crazy gland would not be known until Dr. Rudstad received the pathology report which he would review with me at my follow-up appointment the following week. My type of cancer was confirmed by a pathologist during surgery to be papillary. Dr. Rudstad said this form of cancer is not aggressive in nature and is often referred to as being a "micro cancer."

Dr. Rudstad performed a vocal cord test following surgery and all seemed good. This was news to me as I could not carry a tune if it had a handle on it. Seriously though, as a public speaker, I appreciated knowing that I could continue in that job. The other good news was that no tumors were seen in the lymph nodes and he did not remove my parathyroid. Dr. Rudstad's recommendation was that I did not need radiation, but that the decision would be made in my consultation with Dr. Christensen.

When I was being rolled into my hospital room, I was much more coherent and remember scooting over onto my bed. Lori and a couple of other friends, Pat and Margo, were there waiting to see me. We had nice visits as I settled in and I was surprised how good I felt. I did have some pain but not so much from the incision as from having the breathing tube down my throat. My surgical incision was about two inches long with dissolving stitches followed by a type of "super glue" to prevent infection.

The nurse came in and we immediately connected because he had and appreciated a good sense of humor. I could tell that I was feeling pretty well as I began cracking jokes with him almost immediately. I believed that my illness was not to be taken out on the nurse or any other people or creatures. I needed to be honest about how I was doing but recognize that others have feelings too and I did not need to tromp across them.

The nurse filled me in on what would be happening in terms of meals, getting up and moving around, etc. Depending upon how I was doing, I would stay either one or two nights in the hospital, but I wanted to know what was involved in my being released. Being a to-do list kind of woman, I appreciated finding out the three criteria necessary for my leaving the hospital: 1) I had to feel good, 2) I had to be eating and drinking and 3) my parathyroid had to be absorbing calcium.

The first two steps were interrelated because if I did not feel good, I would not be eating and drinking. In terms of the third step sometimes after the thyroid is removed, the calcium levels can plummet since they are regulated by the thyroid. The goal is to see if the parathyroid has stepped in and absorbed the calcium in the absence of the thyroid.

So I had my first test of the three steps and I failed miserably! The goal was to see how my body would do with absorbing calcium so I was given some pills to take and began drinking liquids as I was pretty thirsty. If that went well, then I would try solid food as soon as possible. After all, I was feeling pretty good or so I thought until I shifted my position in bed.

Lori and Rebecca helped me shift up straighter in bed and then they sat back down. I moved ever so slightly and suddenly felt that feeling like when I had drank too much in my college partying days. Fortunately, I had a clear plastic barf bag next to me and I grabbed it. The good news is that my aim was accurate and I had nothing in my stomach except liquid and the calcium pills. So, the mess was not too bad to clean up.

One of my friends got the nurse who came in to inspect the situation. I handed him the bag and asked if the calcium pills were in there or did I have to take them again. I suspect I was whining a bit as I asked that question.

The nurse's sense of humor kicked in immediately. He held the bag up in mock horror and said, "I'm not looking in there to see if the pills are inside. You're going to have to take them again." Everybody in the room burst out laughing.

He continued "And you're going to have to go onto a clear diet. Water, broth, juice, Jell-o."

"Pudding?" I somewhat innocently suggested.

"Did you hear me say clear?" he said facetiously. I laughed out loud and nodded. He brought me various clear items and I set the goal to keep them down so then I could eat up. Over the course of the next few hours, I drank more broth, juice and water than I had previously done this century.

Throughout the evening, I had a steady stream of visitors and thoroughly enjoyed the company. I am blessed to have amazing people in my life and truly enjoy when I am able to connect my friends and family members who did not know each other. Soon the time passed and late evening had arrived. I said goodnight to the last of my visitors and settled in for the night.

I knew that one of the challenges of being in a hospital is getting enough sleep as nurses had to give me medicine and take vital signs. In addition, I would need to go to the bathroom as the clear diet would clearly need somewhere to go. So I figured out that when the nurse came to do what he had to do that I would use the opportunity to use the restroom. By doing so, I minimized my interruptions and got some pretty good sleep.

The next morning, the visitors started coming early as some friends stopped by on their way to work. Around lunchtime, Stacia came and brought me a prayer journal and special pen for writing in it. She asked how I was doing and we compared notes about being in the hospital. It did my heart good to have her come by and she seemed to enjoy herself as well.

Dr. Rudstad stopped in and checked my tests and incision. He said that I would be released that afternoon. So, I was ahead of schedule as I expected to not be discharged until the next day. I would have done a happy dance but I was rhythmetically challenged enough before the surgery and was pretty sure that had not changed as a result of my thyroidectomy.

Lori's Mom, Judy, came by to take me back to Lori and Mike's home. We gathered up the various cards, books, flowers and other gifts I had received during my short stay as well as the very handy water pitcher and the spare barf bag (because you never know).

TRAUMA CHANGES PEOPLE

Several years ago, I was having dinner with my friend, Lisa, and her barely-teenage daughter, Dove. Lisa is a counselor by profession and I am a counselor in life so we are prone to analyzing situations and how people respond to them. A mutual friend of ours had an unexpected health crisis and several people in his life were doing things that were difficult to explain let alone understand. Lisa and I were discussing what was going on and trying to figure out the responses of these people whose behavior simply left us shaking our heads.

Dove was listening to our conversation without comment as she was focusing on her spaghetti. In between bites, she said three words that have stuck with me ever since: "Trauma changes people". Lisa and I stared at her and then at each other as if to say, "out of the mouth of babes". From that moment on, I refer to that very insightful teenager, now college student, as Dr. Dove.

Well Dr. Dove's insight came home to roost when I began my cancer recovery process. Something about staring death down and death blinking forever changed my perspective on life. However, I wanted to get to that "something" and that meant time for a LOT of self-reflection

As expected and appreciated, Lori, Mike, Bryce and Stacia were amazingly gracious hosts and made me feel right at home. I stayed in the basement and gave them their space as they gave me mine. I joked with Lori that I could tell who was walking across the floor above me by the loudness and pace of their steps.

I rested when I needed to and did other recovery things as well. I really enjoy music so I spent time listening to the broad range of music I like including classical, Christian, rock, Christian rock and other combinations. Reading is also a favorite pastime of mine and I spent many hours lost in books. I had accumulated a stack of volumes to read while I recovered from my surgery and began digging into them. However, the recovery activity I did and enjoyed the most was writing.

From the time I was young, I knew that I loved to write and wanted to pursue my passion as a career. However, I came from a practical family of doctors, lawyers and such so the idea of becoming a writer as a profession seemed out of the question. Because I knew how much I enjoyed writing and that I would not be able to do it for a living, I chose not to do much as a hobby. My reasoning was that I would be upset by not being able to pursue writing so why fan the flame? So, I chose to take another career path starting off thinking I would be an attorney. Actually, my very first career choice was announced to my mom when I was a very small child. I told her I was going to be a pink elephant trainer. Although I had many jobs in the course of my life, that was not one of them.

But writing was where I belonged and a series of family tragedies made me realize that fact. Dad's death, Paul's illness and another family health crisis were my wakeup call. I knew that I did not want to get to the end of my life wishing that I had pursued writing so I decided to immediately quit teaching at Boise State and pursue writing and publishing.

Enter my long-time friend, Kelly, whom I had known since elementary school. Our dads were both engineers and our Moms were 2/3 of the Merry Mother Puppeteers, a trio of women who wrote and performed holiday-themed puppet shows in the elementary schools around Idaho Falls. Our families spent many Thanksgivings together as her dad tried to indoctrinate me to the ways of Oklahoma Sooners football.

Kelly and I went to high school together where we were both in debate. After graduation, Kelly and I ended up studying computer science at the University of Idaho in the early 1980s. Over the years, we stayed in touch including reuniting with other eastern Idaho friends over the Christmas holidays after college.

While I took longer to get my degree and find my career, Kelly immediately used her computer science degree and took a job after college working at Hewlett-Packard. We stayed in touch over the years and I would visit her and her family in Washington State, but the point she came roaring back into my life was when my dad died suddenly.

In July 2006, I was teaching summer school at Boise State University when I received word that Dad was in the hospital. I packed my bags for what was to be a two day visit to see Dad and Mom. I arrived on a Saturday morning and by Sunday evening, Dad was gone. I ended up not going home for another ten days. Physically and emotionally exhausted, I was quite thankful when Kelly called at a particularly trying time. We spent nearly two hours on the phone and she helped me focus on the tasks at hand including good self-care techniques. I know that her advice was a major reason I was able to make it through my Dad's funeral, delivering his eulogy, and the aftermath.

A few weeks later, Kelly called and offered to coach me through the process of getting my first book written and published. At that point, I was working on a book but had no intention of leaving my teaching job at Boise State. On the other hand, Kelly had left her job at HP to focus on being a life coach. Now, I had a basic opinion about life coaching as I believed it was for people who did not have one…a life I mean. Oh how wrong I was about that belief!

I took Kelly up on her offer and she began helping me get the structure and organization necessary to make my book a reality. I was plodding along getting the book put together and contacting publishers when Paul's first brain tumor was diagnosed.

Well I did not need any more reminders that life was too short and regrets too easy. I called Kelly and told her that I was going to quit teaching at BSU and pursue writing and publishing full-time. Like Dr. Dove before her, Kelly uttered very memorable words that have stayed with me to this day: "Jane, make a plan and work that plan."

So with Kelly's help, I did just that. I made the decision that I would teach the spring and fall semesters and summer session of 2007 and then leave to become a full-time author and a publisher. I told nobody but Kelly what I was doing as I did not want the word to accidentally slip out. Just before the fall 2007 semester started, I walked into my boss' office and told her that this would be my last semester. She was a bit surprised but understood as we were friends and she had seen all that I had gone through in the last year.

In December 2007, my dream became a reality as I formed Freundship Press and began writing books as my career. Since writing was now a major focus of my life, I began doing as much of it as I possibly could in as many different facets of my life as possible. I followed the advice of John C. Maxwell in his excellent book "How Successful People Think" and began spending time thinking and capturing my thoughts in a journal. I began writing a blog on a variety of subjects as that would hone my writing skills. However, I found particular benefit in writing as I was trying to deal with struggles or issues.

One of Lori's excellent initial pieces of advice to me after I was diagnosed with cancer was to start a journal. She did not have to twist my arm at all as I had found the therapeutic benefit of getting my thoughts, feelings, beliefs, and ideas out of my heart and my head and down onto paper. Rather than being spiritually, emotionally and mentally constipated, I chose to clean myself out by articulating both through writing and talking.

I should have stock in theme notebooks for as many as I have used and given away in the last several years. So I went to my stash of notebooks and pulled one out to begin journaling about my cancer journey. Each of my notebooks is labeled with such titles as "Thinking Journal", "Reading Journal", "Bible studies" and other subjects. Immediately, I knew what this journal would be titled and so I scrawled the words across the cover: "Eggshells and Elephants".

From the time I arrived at Lori and Mike's house, I began writing to capture my journey and to work through all that was going on in my life. The journal already contained notes from meeting with doctors as well as questions I wanted answered. Those writings became the basis for this book and the next one I am working on regarding my cancer journey. That journal and the self-reflection time I spent have been priceless helping me on my road to recovery and transitioning to my life post-cancer.

However in the midst of staying with the Mers family, I had a rapid crash back to reality. I arrived at their home on Thursday, the day after my surgery with the plan of staying about a week depending upon how I was feeling and what Dr. Rudstad said about my release to being able to drive.

On Sunday, I called the kennel to find out how Moose and Mickey were faring and because I missed them. The fine folks at the facility knew what was going on with my cancer as I had been open with them. We had planned for Moose and Mickey to stay a week but also recognized that such arrangements could change very quickly and they did.

"Something is wrong with Moose," the co-owner of the kennel said. "He just is not himself and is laying down by himself a lot. He is not even playing with Mickey."

Now if those roles had been reversed and Mickey was not doing well, I would not have been too terribly surprised. When Mom was dying at home, Mickey would not go anywhere near her bed. While he was usually a permanent fixture at her feet, Moose filled that role in Mom's last days. I firmly believe that dogs get depressed as Mickey showed when Mom was dying and in the first few months after her death.

But Moose was a different canine in that sense. Although he had challenges like losing his eye, Moose rolled with the punches. After Mom's death, he transitioned quite well from Idaho Falls to Boise. So for Moose to be the one who was down in the dumps did not fit his MO.

"I am going to make arrangements to come get Moose and Mickey and have them stay with a friend. I will come pick them up as soon as I can," I said to the kennel man.

"That is a good idea," he replied. "See you when you get here."

I picked up the phone and called my dear friend, Binkie. God does an incredible job of putting people in our lives at times when we really need them. For me, Binkie was such a person.

Turmoil is an understatement about life after Mom's death and Paul's surgery soon after for the return of his brain tumor. When I came back to Boise in between those two events, I knew I would need some time to transition to life before Moose and Mickey joined my home. I needed a temporary foster home for them with somebody who could appreciate the trauma they had gone through after losing Mom. Mickey had been with my parents from the time he was a puppy until Mom's death when Mickey was almost nine years old.

Thankfully, I am blessed with a terrific network of friends and other contacts so I put them to work (and social media helped out too). I put out the word particularly amongst my animal loving friends and hit pay dirt relatively quickly. My friend Kim had a theater colleague named Helene who was an animal lover like Kim and me. Helene's Mom, Binkie, was in her 80s, and also loved animals. Binkie readily agreed to take Moose and Mickey for a couple of weeks assuming all parties (human and canine) agreed.

From the time the boys and I walked into Binkie's house, we got along quite well. Binkie had a gentle way of talking with the dogs similar to how Mom had done and they relaxed immediately. I was particularly concerned with how Mickey would do and Binkie made him feel right at home.

Binkie also made me feel right at home as we clicked immediately. A devout Catholic, Binkie walked the walk as well as talking the talk. Not only did I see that in her daily life but also in a horrific incident that she and her late husband, Bob, turned into an amazing blessing.

In the mid 1970s, Binkie and Bob's oldest son was living in an apartment in Boise. When she had not heard from him in a few days, Binkie went to their son's apartment and found him dead. He had been murdered by a couple of neighbors who wanted his stereo.

In an incredible act of compassion, Binkie said she sat at the trial and could not wish death upon these two men. Furthermore, she forgave them. The men did not receive the death penalty, but Binkie's Christ-like attitude and behavior did not stop there. She and Bob formed the first chapter of Compassionate Friends in the Boise area and helped countless other parents whose children had been murdered or otherwise died. Talk about making lemonade from lemons!

Dogs have an incredible sense of people and Moose and Mickey knew that Binkie cared for them. That first time I left them with her, Mickey was a bit anxious but quickly settled down. Each time they stayed with Binkie after that, Moose and Mickey were more and more comfortable with her.

When I explained to Binkie that Moose was not doing well and asked if they could stay with her for a few days, she did not hesitate to say, "Yes!" This assistance was above and beyond the call of duty as she had recently adopted a dog, also named Mickey, and the three canines were just getting to know each other. This would be the first time that Moose and my Mickey would be staying with Binkie's Mickey. However, Binkie was good with it and that was what was important to me. I thanked her and said we would be there as soon as possible.

My next call was to my old friend Sonja who was one of my Boundary Buddies. Sonja and I lived in the same dorm at the University of Idaho in the 1980s. I was the first person Sonja met on campus when I knocked on her door and introduced myself (she says I burst into her room). Amazingly, Sonja did not drop out on the spot and we have remained friends over the years.

I explained the Moose and Mickey dilemma and that I needed a ride as Lori was not available to drive me. Like Binkie, Sonja did not hesitate and soon was at the Mers' doorstep to take me to the kennel to get Moose and Mickey and go to Binkie's home.

Moose indeed was not himself when I went to pick him up and although glad to see me, he was not full of his usual energy (however Mickey made up the difference). Moose sat in my lap as Sonja drove to Binkie's house. Once we arrived there, Binkie, Sonja and I spent some time visiting while the dogs sniffed each other's rear ends and did the canine version of getting acquainted. When we left, all three dogs hardly seemed to notice as they were playing together. I breathed a huge sigh of relief.

After Sonja took me back to Lori and Mike's, I settled back into the rest of Sunday with the plan of what the next couple of days would look like. Dr. Rudstad wanted to see me that week while I was not to see Dr. Christensen for about six weeks. Assuming that Dr. Rudstad would give me the go-ahead to drive, I would be able to go back to my home after the appointment. Being a to-do list woman like me, Lori suggested we make a grocery store trip after the Dr. Rudstad appointment if I got clearance to go back home. Sounded like a good idea to me so we planned accordingly.

The follow-up appointment with Dr. Rudstad went well although he had some not too surprising news about the tiny tumors speckled across the bottom of my crazy gland. The pathology report indicated that my peppered pals were cancerous. As a result, he felt that I may need to follow-up with radiation. He saw radiation as a preventative measure to hopefully address any remaining cancer cells in the area where the thyroid was removed and the lymph nodes remained. Dr. Rudstad said that he would do radiation if it were him because it would give him peace of mind. However, he said the radiation decision would be left up to Dr. Christensen and me.

In addition, Dr. Rudstad gave me permission to drive, but recommended that I remain in "recovery mode" for several weeks by resting and taking things easy. He said no straining or lifting. As I had already planned to take the month of December off to recover physically, mentally, emotionally and spiritually, his words sounded very good to me.

So Lori and I went from Dr. Rudstad's office to the grocery store where I purchased food to restock my fridge and feed my animals. We went back to her home and loaded up her car with my stuff for the trip to my house. Then, we sat at her counter syncing up our schedules for the next week. I had a brainstorm!

"I know Dr. Christensen's office said to wait six weeks to come in, but why don't I call them and see if they would see me earlier." Lori agreed and I dialed the number.

That phone call brought home the lesson that a lot of information was coming and going through my cancer journey and that communication is very important. Anyway, the nurse explained that I needed to come in to see the doctor that week and was not supposed to wait for six weeks. In addition, I was to start a low iodine diet immediately and then have radiation in two weeks.

I explained that I thought whether I had RAI (radiation) was a decision that was not yet made. She informed me that I was incorrect and began telling me what was involved in a low iodine diet. Of course, the foods were those I had just purchased at the grocery store.

As I thought about the two week timeframe, I knew that I would have to find boarding for all my dogs and cats as I could not be around them while I was taking radiation. Two weeks put the dates as right in between Christmas and New Years. I had a better chance of getting struck by lightning than finding kennel space for all five pets that week on such short notice.

My head was reeling as I hung up the phone and explained to Lori what I had just been told. As we talked about the options, I had a moment of clarity and said to Lori: "I refuse to make a decision on this from a point of panic. I am going to talk with the doctor, see what he says and then make my radiation decision." After all, the cancer was very slow growing and if RAI was needed, doing so immediately was not necessary. Lori agreed.

I was not going to let this issue RAI-n on my parade. Trauma had changed me and I was looking forward to discovering even more about myself.

NEW NORMAL

After I got home, I took a day to rest and unpack before I went to pick up Moose and Mickey from Binkie's house. I had made an appointment with my vet to have her see if anything was wrong with Moose's health. Her examination revealed two very important pieces of information. First, Moose is losing sight in his remaining eye. That news was not particularly surprising but the other piece certainly was a shock: Moose is showing signs of "Doggy Alzheimer's". I did not know that dogs could get Alzheimer's, but then again, I never knew that cats could get AIDS until Curtis was diagnosed with the Feline AIDS Virus. Incidentally, Curtis' FIV diagnosis was 10 years ago and he has no signs of the disease affecting him.

The vet explained that Moose likely felt out of routine when he was at the kennel as there was a lot going on. Between the loss of eyesight and surroundings he had not been in for quite a while, the kennel setting was just too much.

I told her that I had noticed Moose licking Mickey a lot more which the latter did not appreciate. The vet said that by licking Mickey, Moose could keep track of where he was and would not feel lost. She gave me a pill to give both dogs when they got anxious and suggested giving both Moose and Mickey even more love and attention. The latter was easier than the former as sometimes three people are needed to give Mickey a pill (another vet refers to him as "the Devil Dog").

The other doctor's appointment after my first few days back was for me. Lori came along with me to see Dr. Christensen. We talked about radiation and such factors as the cancer showing no signs of spreading and an increased risk of some other health problems in people who have had RAI. I explained that having radiation was not on my "Bucket List". Furthermore, it sounded like to me that my having RAI would be like using a sledgehammer to kill a fly that may or may not be there. In the end, I opted to not have radiation and Dr. Christensen agreed. The weather forecast of RAI-n on my parade had been cancelled!

Dr. Christensen said that I was otherwise healing well and that the next challenge was to get my synthetic thyroid balanced. This would involve regular blood tests and adjusting the dosage accordingly. Otherwise, I was to come back for a follow-up appointment in six months.

Given that my recovery from the surgery was going so well and that I did not know any better, I thought getting my synthetic thyroid balanced would be just as easy. Well, I booked an immediate passage to Fantasy Island with that belief as the truth which turned out to be much different! I had never imagined that the process of getting my synthetic thyroid balanced would take so very long, but fortunately, I had a skill that helped make the process a bit easier: I am a self-admitted research geek.

Over the course of my college career, I took seven research classes or internships. I remember talking to another student about taking a communication research methods class as an elective. She looked at me with a very puzzled look and said, "Haven't you ever heard of bowling?"

Well, I put my research passion to use and started finding out as much as I possibly could about living without my thyroid. My research focus prior to surgery had been to learn as much as I could about thyroid cancer and radiation. I had not even thought about what life would be like after my surgery because once I realized I did not have to have radiation. I thought I was pretty much in the clear in terms of any long-term issues. Oh how wrong I was!

The first big surprise was my foggy brain. I was stunned that I would have trouble remembering information and doing mental tasks. I have a talent for doing arithmetic in my head to the extent that some of my friends call me "Jane Man" (think "Rain Man", the movie starring Dustin Hoffman and Tom Cruise). After my thyroidectomy, I had difficulty doing basic addition in my head.

The second stunner was the change (albeit temporary) in my immune system. Prior to my thyroidectomy, I rarely if ever caught a cold and cannot remember the last time I had the flu. In the few months after my surgery, I caught more colds than Willie Mays caught fly balls (although I thankfully managed to avoid catching the flu).

Another challenge I faced is adapting my lifestyle so that certain strategies could replace the operation of my now dearly departed thyroid. However figuring out those strategies has not been easy. No doctor, nurse, other health care professional or single individual has handed me the answers on a silver platter. In fact, I have had to not only figure out what functions were missing but also how to replace them once I identified them.

Enter a couple of my friends who could relate to what I was going through. Although neither had had thyroid cancer, each had issues with malfunctioning thyroids. I had coffee, conversations and other communication with them to learn as much as I could about what I was facing. They taught me a great deal about alternative treatments and turned me onto very helpful resources. One book in particular turned out to be very useful to me as I figured out how to proceed.

The book was one I mentioned earlier and was written by Mary Shomon. The book is titled "Living Well With Hypothyroidism:

What Your Doctor Does not Tell You...That You Need to Know" Shomon's book opened my eyes to so much I had never considered about the thyroid and adapting to lack of one. Although the book was not about thyroid cancer specifically, I knew that many of the principles applied to people who had any issues with the function of their thyroids.

The first strategy I learned was that synthetic thyroid should not be taken within four hours of calcium or iron. I knew that I should wait an hour after taking my medicine before eating but did not know the calcium and iron limitation. I would take my synthetic thyroid in the morning but was beginning to consider altering that timeframe.

Weight gain can also be an issue with thyroid problems. Although my other health numbers were always good, I have struggled with weight since I was young. Although my good cholesterol could be a bit better, my blood pressure and other crucial health figures were well within acceptable range despite my extra weight. Regardless, I knew that I felt better when I was not heavy so one of my goals was to reduce my weight.

Well, having no thyroid can make weight loss a problem, but I read in Shomon's book that a good way to jump start my metabolism was to have 25% of my protein in my breakfast meal. The problem with that idea was that my protein often came in the form of cheese, yogurt and other calcium rich foods.

That's when I decided to start taking my synthetic thyroid at night so that not only would I ensure I did not eat for an hour afterward, but I could also get the necessary proteins as part of breakfast. The results paid off and I immediately began to lose weight.

Another really good decision I made was to become active in the LiveSTRONG program at the YMCA. The program met twice a week for eight weeks and included diet, exercise and other lifestyle changes for people adapting to life after cancer. Lori had become aware of the program through Stacia's cancer and encouraged me to get involved. A long-time Y member, I was a bit surprised that I had not heard of the program before. I knew about LiveSTRONG itself as I am a sports fan and heard about Lance Armstrong's battle with cancer and his formation of the LiveSTRONG foundation.

I arrived for the first day of the class and found a mixture of men and women with various stories to tell about single or multiple battles with cancer. While I knew they had had tougher cancer journeys than I did, I knew that mine was still important because it was happening to me. I could and would still be concerned about helping them, but my main responsibility was to "put on my own oxygen mask first" and focus on my recovery. I would not do others any good if I did not take care of myself.

Our group leaders, Vicki and Mark, are very good at what they do. Their tricky job was to find the balance between compassion and gentle pushing to get us to meet our health goals. We walked, lifted weights, did yoga, stretched and used some equipment that bared a strong resemblance to a medieval torture device. We also shared stories, struggles and suggestions. Something about being in a room filled with kindred spirits twice a week made adjusting to the new normal a bit easier.

The LiveSTRONG program reminded me of the importance of incorporating exercise, eating right, drinking plenty of water and taking care of myself. Most importantly, LiveSTRONG emphasized what Shomon's book had made clear: living life post cancer meant thinking outside the box as no one source had all of the answers. I had to adapt my life physically, mentally, socially, spiritually and emotionally. Oh how vital that realization became as I faced another unexpected health issue soon after!

MARCH ON BY

Technology is a tool I use in many aspects of my life although I am not a latest and greatest kind of techie. I did not get a cell phone until about five years ago and a laptop did not become part of my repertoire until about three years ago, but one change I have NOT made is to an electronic calendar.

When I was in college, I discovered the desktop paper calendar and I have been a happy camper ever since. Visuals are important as they help me to remember important things and a desktop calendar helps me to see the big picture. My life history can be greatly understood by my calendar as that is how I track my time.

Speaking of which, as time marched on I could not see the forest for the trees of my new normal. I was spending a great deal of time focusing on where I was and not so much looking to moving forward. Identifying such ruts for oneself can be very difficult and admitting it an even bigger step. Fortunately for me, Lori stepped in and spoke the "truth in love".

After I responded to a "how are you?" e-mail from her, she wrote me back a very carefully worded e-mail with a very simple question: "What about asking your doctor about an anti-depressant?" I thought about what she said but probably for not as long as I should have.

I had no problem talking about what I was thinking and feeling so the idea that I was depressed seemed out of the realm of possibility for me. The reality I did not want to face is that the word "depression" had a long-term and deep meaning to me and the possibility that I was depressed scared me.

From the time I was in elementary school, I saw first-hand the impact depression had on my family as Dad was chronically depressed. Over the course of his life, Dad had two nervous breakdowns. I remember visiting Dad in the hospital during those breakdowns which occurred in my junior high and high school years.

As I researched my own cancer, I read a great deal about the link between the thyroid and depression. If a thyroid is not functioning correctly, depression is a common occurrence. The thyroid-depression connection light bulb came on when I realized Dad had undiagnosed slow growing thyroid cancer for many years. No wonder he was so depressed because the true source of his problem was not being treated.

I would like to say that once Dad's thyroid cancer was treated that he ended up being depression free, but in fact the opposite happened. His doctor was having his own health issues and nobody seemed to be keeping good track of Dad's synthetic thyroid levels. One doctor thought another one was taking care of it, but in a classic case of Everybody thought Somebody was doing it but Nobody was, Dad's levels were way out of whack.

Now having gone through my own thyroid cancer battle, I have a much better understanding of what was happening with Dad. I specifically remember the summer of 2000 when I would spend hours talking with him and he would tell me that the ceiling was caving in or some other illogical event was occurring. No matter how many times I tried to reason with my very logical father that the ceiling was not caving in, Dad did not believe me.

One week, in what was a very difficult but very necessary move, Mom and Paul took Dad to a mental hospital in Pocatello for treatment. I have amazing amounts of respect for Mom and Paul for encouraging Dad to get the help and for Dad, through his brain fog, for realizing he needed the help. At the mental hospital, the doctors ran a blood test and determined Dad's synthetic thyroid levels were out of whack. They changed his dosage and Dad was back home in less than a week and on his way to recovery. Although he struggled with depression for the rest of his life, the problem was never as bad as it had been prior to his visit to the Pocatello hospital.

But despite what I knew about depression and thyroid from both personal and book experience, I did not want to face the reality that I might be depressed. So, I decided to ride on the USS Denial for at least a while. However, that ship would soon come into port.

In April 2012, I made the decision to switch the management of my synthetic thyroid to Dr. Nona. I knew that menopause would be coming for a very long visit to my life anytime. So, having one doctor oversee all of my medicines made the most sense to me. For the most part, I choose female doctors who are about my age as they face the same kind of health issues as I do when I do. Also, they usually laugh at my culturally-age-related humor. Dr. Nona fit both categories.

Several years ago, I attended a women's church retreat and ended up banging my head on a post in the middle of the night. I did not have my glasses on and walked right into the beam as I am blind as a bat without my spectacles. A week later when I could not remember simple words like basket, I made an appointment to have my head examined.

I began explaining my problem to Dr. Nona. "I came out of the grocery store and could not find my car."

"Jane," she replied. "That happens to me all the time." We had a good laugh and then I went for tests that showed I did have a slight concussion.

On the morning of my first appointment with Dr. Nona to manage my synthetic thyroid, I was laying in bed thinking about my day. As I thought about what Lori had said about depression and thinking about my family medical history, the reality hit me in the face. Depression has both an emotional/mental and a physical component. My willingness to talk and share helped with the emotional/mental component, but I was doing very little to deal with the physical component. My body needed help and an anti-depressant could do that. So when I had my appointment that day, I asked Dr. Nona about going on an anti-depressant while I got my synthetic thyroid balanced and she said yes.

At that point, the lesson I learned from Mary Shomon's book and the LiveSTRONG program intersected with how Dad approached his own depression. He knew that the treatment involved cognitive, physical and emotional aspects. A pill was not and did not solve his depression, but he used a multi-faceted approach. Dad worked on changing his thinking about depression and researched as much as he could on the subject. He ate healthy, exercised regularly and took his medicine ever day. Also, Dad talked about how he was feeling thus hitting the emotional part of his depression head on.

So I figuratively threw Shomon, LiveSTRONG and Dad's methods into a box and added a spiritual component for good measure and came up with my own ways for dealing with my depression. I altered my diet to compensate for the lack of a thyroid and the presence of depression. One such strategy is to drink a lot of water which helps keep my system flushed out. I exercise regularly and pray even more frequently. Finally, I put my research geekiness to work and stay current as much as I can with what is happening in the worlds of thyroid cancer and depression. However, I take care to not get too much information as that can be overwhelming and counterproductive as well as resulting in more depression.

As I began feeling better, I got more into my usual routine and made a very interesting discovery. One day soon after I started the anti-depressant, I was sitting at my desk and was surprised to discover that I had not switched my desktop calendar past February. Since the month was now April, I turned the page and was even more startled to discover that the month of March was totally blank. I had not recorded a single activity on my calendar. The truth of my depression was staring me right in the face. The month had Marched on by and I had not even noticed. Not going to let that happen again.

LESSONS LEARNING

As I bring this book to a close, I am no longer taking an anti-depressant and have my thyroid levels in good balance after almost eight months. So as I end this portion of my cancer journey, looking at lessons learning seems like an appropriate way to transition to the next chapter of my life. Notice that I do not speak in the past but rather the present tense as this is an ongoing process. In fact, I am learning so much that I am writing another book just on the lessons cancer is teaching me.

Speaking of which, the lessons are falling into several categories with the first one being about me. For example, my cancer journey is teaching me a change in priorities. For example, when I stared death down and death blinked, having to wait a few extra minutes in line does not seem all that problematic. I use the time to pray or take a few deep breaths. Speaking of breathing, my cancer journey has breathed new life into my walk with the Lord and I am particularly excited by those lessons.

The importance of education is also getting hammered into my head. As I have stressed throughout this book, I believe in learning but my cancer journey has focused that education process. For instance, I am learning and preaching as much as possible is to get your family medical history researched and into one document. As I mentioned before, Dr. Nona told me that having my family medical history in her hands is what prompted her to order the Tg test that resulted in my cancer diagnosis.

If not for that family medical history, I may not have found out that I had cancer.

Furthermore, you would be staring right now at a blank page as I would not have written this book. Seriously though, go to the Freundship Press YouTube channel. You will find a video I have made on how to compile a family medical history. The process is not as difficult as you might think and every bit of information you can get will help out. If you don't feel like searching, then use this link to get to the video: http://www.youtube.com/watch?v=sxFGw-Lre6s.

The other category of lessons I am learning are about life itself. Life is not a parade to watch go by or a performance to view but rather a reality to be lived. For each and every one of us, the reality called life takes a unique form and lasts for a different amount of time.

Tim McGraw summed it up so well in his song "Live Like You Were Dying" as he pointed out the importance of living for what really matters. But here's the truth that few people want to face: we are all dying. Some of us are fortunate enough to find that reality out and be given another chance to live. I pray that your "A-HA" moment is so real that you wake up and live like you were dying. What is stopping you from doing so right now?

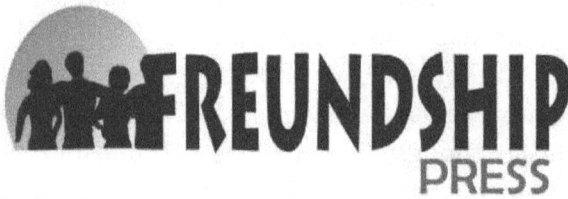

FREUNDSHIP PRESS

Positively influencing lives through friendship, communication, and education.

PO Box 9171

Boise, ID 83707

208-407-7457

info@freundshippress.com

www.freundshippress.com

In addition, Jane Freund and
Freundship Press can be found on
Facebook, Twitter, LinkedIn, Pinterest,
Google+ and smoke signals.
OK, we're joking about
the smoke signals...